Leadership Development for Nurses and Midwives

Leadership Development for Nurses and Midwives

Edited by

GEMMA STACEY, PhD, MN, RN, PGCHE, PFHEA
Florence Nightingale Foundation

GRETA WESTWOOD, CBE, PhD, MSc, RN
Florence Nightingale Foundation

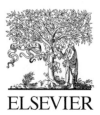

ELSEVIER

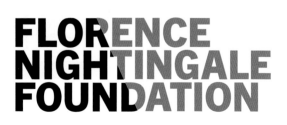

FLORENCE
NIGHTINGALE
FOUNDATION

ISBN: 978-0-3238-7049-8

Content Strategist: Robert Edwards
Content Project Manager: Shubham Dixit
Design: Ryan Cook
Marketing Manager: Samantha Page

Printed in India.

Last digit is the print number: 9   8   7   6   5   4   3   2   1

CONTENTS

In my career as a nurse and midwifery leader, I have had the privilege of holding the positions of chief nursing officer (CNO) for Wales, Scotland, and later England. Whilst chair of the World Health Organisation's Global Advisory Group on Nursing in Geneva, I helped ensure that strong nursing resolutions were passed by the World Health Assembly. Whilst I remain so proud of all these achievements, I am most proud of my current role as chair of the Florence Nightingale Foundation (FNF).

The FNF enables nurses and midwives to realise the confidence to become the very best leaders, not just in the United Kingdom but across the world. The FNF seeks to inspire its community of alumni to have significant influence through the skills they developed during their scholarships and leadership programmes. I benefited from a similar development opportunity in my early career which enabled me to meet people I wouldn't have usually met, but most importantly, it opened my eyes to what was possible. Before the programme, I wanted to be the best ward sister in the country, but after this experience, I wanted to be the best CNO in the world. This is what I am hoping this book will fire up in every one of you.

We have designed this book in the same way we design our leadership programmes and scholarships. We take the approach that every nurse and midwife is a leader and holds leadership attributes. What you may not yet have is a strong sense of your personal leadership signature – the unique way in which you will influence practice and develop your teams to perform at the very best of their ability. We understand the personal and professional barriers which can prevent nurses and midwives from achieving this level of influence, and this book aims to help you to navigate through those barriers. Some of this will be about developing your confidence, self-awareness, and personal presence, and others will be about understanding the political context of your work and the cultural constraints you must become aware of in order to challenge.

I would like to share with you two pieces of advice that I hope will inspire you to view this book as the start of a journey to a career path that has no limits. The first is to find your heroes. I will tell you about three people who have inspired me. All three have been achieved against the odds.

The first one, of course, is Florence Nightingale. I am inspired by how she became this legend, how she became such an influence, and how she had the courage to walk the corridors of power to bring about change. She did this by using data. She recognised how crucial it was to build a case for change that is strongly underpinned by the foundation of evidence. What I draw most from her, though, is her empathy. She empathised with individual people, families, the poor, and the disadvantaged. She was alongside them to understand their needs. It was this empathy that gave her the motivation, tenacity, and drive to gather evidence to make change happen. I believe this empathy is within all of us, and we must always recall and pay attention to it as we advance in our leadership positions.

My second inspiration was a nurse who grew up in a small village in Botswana. As a child, she had no access to education and lived in poverty. She was dedicated to educating herself so she could become a nurse. She wanted more than anything to care for others; she wanted to do something to heal the sickness and death that surrounded her. She achieved this against all odds. In the early 1960s, she accessed nurse education in Edinburgh and then Canada but then came back to Botswana where she lobbied the government to set up nursing as a profession. This took years of great struggles, but with huge tenacity, she achieved it and is now known as the mother of nursing in Botswana. Her name was Serara Segarona Kupe Mogwe. I met her 2 years ago in Thailand; she was our Nurse of the Year at the age of 91. The worldwide media surrounded her, and she was so strong and still battling for nursing to be supported and developed further in her home country. If I felt, as I did so often as CNO, that I was making no progress with ministers, I thought of her and her struggles. I reminded myself that if Serara could achieve what she did in her country and never give up, then I should keep going.

My third hero is not a nurse; she was a woman from a very modest background who was determined to travel to space. She fought, within a man's world, to achieve her goal at a time when no women were astronauts. Her name is Helen Sharman, and I had the privilege of meeting her at a conference I hosted as CNO for nurse leaders. The words I most remember from her speech were 'Reach for the stars, go for it!'

The second piece of advice I would like to share with you before you engage with the materials in this book is to discover and foster talent around you. I am most inspired when I have helped to nurture and develop people around me. Ultimately my ambition has always been to enable others in my team and networks to be better than me. My hope is that they will be able to take roles even more senior and influence with even further reach. When I see success in others, I feel immense pride and am reassured that my profession that I love so dearly will be safe in their hands.

I urge you to recognise that it is a privilege to be a nurse or a midwife and that we are all leaders. We have a responsibility to our communities and our teams to role-model the same attributes I have described in my heroes: tenacity, resilience, dedication, and mostly, great courage. To achieve this, we must be inspired by our heroes and nurture the talent among us.

Dame Yvonne Moores

AUTHOR BIOS

Gemma Stacey

Professor Gemma Stacey is a registered mental health nurse and director of academy at the Florence Nightingale Foundation. She leads an extensive programme of commissioned leadership development, policy thought leadership, and applied research which aims to elevate the authority and influence of nursing and midwifery. Her personal research and practice has focused on psychologically safe spaces for health care workers which promote transformational learning, wellbeing, and patient safety. She is a widely published academic author and is committed to supporting novice writers to find their voice to disseminate their expertise.

Greta Westwood

Professor Greta Westwood is a registered nurse and chief executive officer of the Florence Nightingale Foundation (FNF). The Foundation has transformed under her leadership. She established the FNF Academy, providing exclusive and competitive leadership development opportunities for hundreds of nurses and midwives across the career pathway. The Academy also provides thought leadership and policy development to raise the voice of nursing and midwifery. Her clinical practice and research developed the role of genetic nurses across the United Kingdom and laterally with clinical academic nurses and midwives. Greta is an FNF alumna and a 2012 Leadership Scholar. She was awarded the honour of Commander of the Order of the British Empire (CBE) by the Queen in 2021 for services to nursing and midwifery.

Pippa Gough

Pippa Gough has a background in nursing, health visiting, policy development, and research. She was director of policy at the Royal College of Nursing (RCN) and later senior faculty at the King's Fund. She currently works as a coach with both individuals and teams at senior and executive levels. She is highly experienced in designing, commissioning, and facilitating innovative leadership and organisational development programmes within the public sector. She has written widely on nursing, policy, and leadership and is a published poet and author of short stories.

Amy Hart

Amy Hart has been running her own consultancy for over 11 years which specialises in individual, team, and organisational development. Amy holds an MSc in people and organisational development and is fellow of the Chartered Institute of Personnel and Development (CIPD). Prior to running her own consultancy, Amy held numerous senior leader and board positions in the NHS. Amy currently works with many NHS, charitable sector, and private sector organisations regionally, nationally, and internationally. More recently, Amy has set up a company with a partner to provide at-scale interventions for teams within the NHS. Amy's particular area of interest is developing leaders in the NHS that create compassionate, creative, sustainable workplaces.

Catherine Eden

Catherine Eden has 25 years' experience of working at all levels of UK politics including local government, Westminster, the charity sector, and the European Parliament. She also worked in the NHS as a manager. Since 2010, she has run a company that works with leaders in all sectors to help them better understand the politics that affect them and their sector. Much of that work is within the health sector, often helping nurse leaders to navigate the politics and think through how they can be more influential locally and nationally. She has worked with the Florence Nightingale Foundation delivering politics courses since 2010.

Clair Henry

Claire Henry, MBE, is a registered nurse, visiting researcher at the University of Cambridge Palliative and End of Life Care research group, visiting fellow at the Open University coach, and mentor and an independent consultant in health and care. She has worked predominately in palliative and end-of-life care leading national implementation and quality improvement programmes and is committed to supporting health and care staff to use quality improvement to make a difference to patient and family care.

Jane Dwelly

Jane Dwelly is vice president international at CHIME – the College of Healthcare Information Management Executives. In this role Jane directs CHIME's global work to network digital health leaders, deliver digital health education, and accredit senior leaders. Jane leads all digital health training at the Florence Nightingale Foundation and is the programme director for the Digital Health Leadership Academy for Nurses and Midwives. She also leads CHIME's contribution to the digital health curricula on master's courses at the University of Limerick and the University of Wales, Trinity Saint David. Jane was appointed as a trustee of the Florence Nightingale Museum of International Nursing in 2021.

Jonathan Guy Lewis

Jonathan Guy Lewis works extensively as an actor, writer, director, teacher, mentor, and coach and has won a number of awards for his work. An ex-army scholar, he has a degree from Exeter University in Politics & Society and is a graduate from the Guildhall School of Music and Drama. He has had considerable experience over the last 25 years delivering personal development and impact skills training to the corporate world. He specialises in helping leaders understand authentic performance as an aspect of communication and leadership, focusing particularly on how to create and embody trust and confidence while overcoming fear, stress, and anxiety. He has worked all over the globe and has spent several years creating his unique blend of content, performance and forum theatre, immersive role play, improvisation, and creativity master classes. He is the artistic director of the Soldiers' Arts Academy, a platform that engages the military and veteran community in the healing power of creativity. He is also an honorary fellow at Edinburgh University (Nursing Studies).

Susanna C. Shouls

Susanna Shouls is an expert in quality improvement and measurement for improvement methodologies and has considerable experience in programme and project management. She has specific interest in palliative and end-of-life care, patient safety, public health, community development, and same-day emergency care. Susanna has led health economy–wide quality improvement programmes, conducted independent evaluations and research, and designed and worked in a range of national improvement programmes. She is currently working independently for a range of organisations including social services, hospitals, and charities. She has a first degree in human biology and a master's degree in operational research.

The Florence Nightingale Foundation has an established and outstanding reputation for providing leadership development to nurses and midwives (you can learn more about our history in Chapter 1). If you encounter an alumnus of the Florence Nightingale Foundation, they are likely to tell you about the profound personal impact the experience had on their perception of themselves and, as a consequence, their career progression. For example, Barbara Makunde told us, 'I see continuous growth in myself and will grab every opportunity that comes my way. My journey has only just begun with the Florence Nightingale Foundation'. Thousands of others share similar statements which demonstrate the personal and professional impact of their development opportunity with the Foundation.

This book benefits from the insights and perspectives of the range of experts who contribute to our unique approach to leadership development. Reading this book requires you to engage in reflective learning throughout by applying the content of the book to your own context and personal development needs. The approach we adopt is not bound by a rigid set of leadership theories or behaviours. We emphasise the uniqueness of you as a leader. The book will enable you to explore a range of perspectives which will challenge you to enhance your leadership attributes by building confidence and stepping into your authority. Our authors are writing from a position of experience, as they have all worked with nurses and midwives over many years. They each have their own approach and distinctive style which we hope you find engaging and thought-provoking.

The book begins with an introduction to Florence Nightingale and the Foundation. In this chapter, Greta Westwood demonstrates how Florence's passion to improve the experience of people in need of care motivated her to take action with local and international impact. Florence was acutely aware of her privilege and the opportunities this offered her. She exploited her position, utilised her networks, and generated evidence to hold the authority she needed to make a difference. It is these qualities that we hope to foster in our Florence Nightingale Foundation alumni as we enable them to identify their sphere of influence and step into their authority.

Chapter 2 begins this journey by enabling you to explore how your personality preferences influence your approach to leadership and your performance in teams. Our authors, Greta Westwood and Gemma Stacey, emphasise the importance of self-awareness, emotional intelligence, and the investment in reflection and feedback to continuously grow as an authentic leader. In this chapter, we draw upon an evidence-based framework, the Myers–Briggs Type Indicator (MBTI), to enable you to explore your own and team behaviours to maximise on leadership strengths.

The premise of emotional intelligence is built upon in Chapter 3, which focuses on the performance skills required to have presence and impact. In this chapter, Jonathan Guy Lewis (Royal Academy of Dramatic Arts) starts with a focus on confidence and encourages you to consider the psychological and physiologic factors which impact your ability to deliver your message with conviction and assert your expertise in a range of settings, from multidisciplinary team meetings to conference presentations. Lewis offers strategies to enhance your confidence and your presence which draw upon tested approaches used every day in the acting world. This chapter acknowledges that leadership may require us to work outside of our comfort zone if we are to have the impact that we desire. However, with a commitment to practice, rehearsal, and feedback, we are all capable of fostering the skills to have our voice heard.

Chapter 4 considers the concept of psychological safety, which refers to an environment where team members feel able to take interpersonal risks. Pippa Gough shares with you a strategy to promote psychological safety through peer group coaching. This approach to Peer group coaching involves asking powerful open questions to encourage each other to share experiences and explore alternative perspectives. The ability to create psychological safety in teams is a core leadership attribute and is increasingly seen as the consistent factor which defines a working environment where staff feel valued, empowered, and energised. Unsurprisingly this results in better outcomes relating to patient safety and satisfaction. Gough suggests that as leaders we should be investing in strategies to enhance psychological safety by role-modelling and embedding a coaching culture.

Chapter 5 is an extension of this theme. It acknowledges that leadership in health and social care will require consideration of the anxious times in which we are living. In this chapter, Amy Hart explores the impact that anxiety can have on individual and team behaviours. She offers strategies to validate and attend to the emotional impact of our working worlds, with a goal of further enhancing the psychological safety of the environment.

In the next section, we move our attention to the leadership attributes required to influence and manage change. In Chapter 6, Catherine Eden explores this from a political perspective and urges nurses and midwives to exercise political acumen. Catherine demonstrates how nurses are and have always been political influencers at a local, national, and international level; however, we rarely consider our sphere of influence in this way.

We progress this theme through the lens of quality improvement (QI). In Chapter 7, Claire Henry and Susanna Shouls describe the theory and practice of applied QI with several practical examples to illustrate the ways nurses and midwives can lead change and impact the experience of people receiving our services. With some simple tools, underpinned by implementation science, we can leverage this change and measure the impact in cycles of continued improvement. Our alumni often describe this framework as offering them a language to justify and articulate the need for change, offering them confidence to engage key stakeholders.

Chapter 8 applies these principles to the important area of digital transformation. It is now evident that nurses and midwives are becoming increasingly influential in the development and implementation of digital solutions. Jane Dwelley emphasises that this is not about IT technical knowledge, but it is the unique expertise that nurses and midwives bring to understanding the care pathway and as a result understanding how technology can enhance this process. The key is engagement with the wider workforce so that digital solutions are embedded and received with enthusiasm not scepticism. Nurses and midwives are uniquely placed to actively inform communications and education surrounding digital transformation to ensure that the art of health care practice remains at the heart of any digitally enhanced practice.

Chapter 9, our final chapter, emphasises the importance of disseminating our knowledge and expertise through endeavours such as writing for publication. This is conceptualised as a core leadership attribute rarely realised within our profession, even among our most prominent leaders. In this chapter, Gemma Stacey acknowledges the psychological and practical barriers encountered by nurses and midwives which deter them from these activities. Gemma suggests that exploring our individual motivation to write is core to finding the energy and space to prioritise this activity. By the end of the chapter, we hope you feel compelled to share your expertise and demonstrate the central role nurses and midwives have in driving clinical excellence through the publication of your work.

We conclude our book with some final reflections and messages to you as leaders of care, environments, people, services, policies, education, research, and innovation. The recognition of your leadership attributes and investment in your development is central to our purpose as a charity. We continue Florence Nightingale's legacy through the support of your development and the power of creating networks for you to influence and step into your authority as a collective voice. We hope you find this book the first step on this journey and revisit it as your sphere of influence grows beyond any limits that have previously been defined by you or for you.

Gemma Stacey
Greta Westwood

CHAPTER 1

Florence Nightingale and Her Legacy Today

Greta Westwood

> *For us who Nurse, our Nursing is a thing, which, unless in it we are making progress every year, every month, every week, take my word for it we are going back. The more experience we gain, the more progress we can make. The progress you make in your year's training with us is as nothing to what you must make every year after your year's training is over. (May 1872 letter to the probationer-nurses, Nightingale Training School, St Thomas' Hospital, London.)*

CHAPTER OUTLINE

A short history of Florence Nightingale's life and her route into nursing

Her achievements, her leadership attributes, and her relevance today

A history of the Florence Nightingale Foundation and its current work

There are many texts available on her life and particularly her work during the Crimean War, but of course Florence's work continued until she died in 1910. Her legacy continues with the work of the Florence Nightingale Foundation.

OBJECTIVES

To understand
- Florence's family background
- Florence's drive and desire to become a nurse
- Florence's lifetime achievements
- Florence's impact on modern day nursing
- The history and work of the Florence Nightingale Foundation

Florence's Early Life and Her Route to Nursing

This section will describe Florence's family background, her home life, her 'calling', her attempts to become a nurse and her nursing role before the Crimean War.

FAMILY BACKGROUND

Florence was born in Florence, Italy, on 12 May 1820 during her family's European tour. Her sister, Parthenope, was born a year earlier, in Naples, during the same tour. The Nightingale family was a wealthy English family. Florence's father, William Shore, inherited a large lead mining fortune from his maternal great uncle, Peter Nightingale of Lea Hurst, Derbyshire, England. Florence's mother's father, William Smith, was an abolitionist and liberal Member of Parliament (MP) for 46 years. One of her mother's sisters, Joanna, married John Carter, also an MP who later became John Bonham Carter. Their son Henry had a son Walter Bonham Carter, also a liberal MP who married Violet Asquith, the daughter of Lord Asquith, the Prime Minister during the First World War. One of their four children was Raymond, Helena Bonham Carter's father.

Henry Bonham Carter (1827–1921) was the secretary of the Nightingale Fund. A public meeting was held in London at the end of 1855 to recognise the work of Florence Nightingale in Crimea. A £44,039 (equivalent to £3m in 2021) was raised in her honour through public subscriptions, concerts, and other fundraising activities, and soldiers who had fought in the war gave a day's pay. Henry also oversaw the management of the Nightingale Training School at St Thomas's Hospital, London. The Fund has always been safeguarded by the Bonham Carters and is now managed by Helena's brother, **Thomas,** together with a relative of Parthenope's husband's family, Sir Edmund Verney, of Claydon House, Buckinghamshire, England.

FAMILY LIFE

Parthenope and Florence were very different. Parthenope was happy to entertain herself with needlework and sketching whilst Florence concentrated and immersed herself in her studies. Originally both Nightingale sisters were schooled at home by a governess but later, when Florence was 11, they were tutored by their father. They learnt Latin, Greek, Italian, and French, and they studied chemistry, geography, physics, grammar and philosophy. He instructed a maths tutor, John Rickman, one of the creators of the British census, to sent them the Derbyshire's 1832 census return. Florence's love of data and the inspiration for her work as a sanitary reformer may have begun at this time.

The family lived between two homes, Lea Hurst in Derbyshire and Embley Park in Hampshire, the latter for the winter months. It is well documented that Florence lived an unhappy life at home. She was frustrated with the prospect of a privileged Victorian woman's life: married, household manager whilst entertaining her husband's guests, reading, letter writing, and needlework. She came to realise that women were not able to undertake work that was truly worthwhile and rewarding, or indeed they were unable to study to an elite level. She came to see her home as a prison and prompted her work for the emancipation of women.

A favoured distraction from the mundane existence were the visits she made with her female family members to the poor houses in the villages of both homes. She attended to sick relatives and tenants of the family estates. As part of a liberal Unitarian family, Florence found great comfort in her religious beliefs. At the age of 16, at the Hampshire family home, she experienced one of several 'calls from God'. She viewed her calling as reducing human suffering. Nursing seemed the suitable route to serve both God and humankind. She even refused a marriage proposal from Richard Monkton Milnes as she chose to stay single to better serve God and society.

Hospitals at that time were dirty and unhygienic and staffed by 'nurses' who were often drunk. A nurse's work was viewed as being a servant or a cleaner. Florence decided a new kind of nurse was needed, a nurse that was formally trained in hygiene, efficiency, and organisation. Once she decided she wanted to become a nurse, she set about planning this route. She was friends with a physician at Salisbury Infirmary, Wiltshire, England, and secured a 3-month nurse training programme there. Her parents were horrified and refused her to follow her calling. To be a nurse was deemed by her family as an inappropriate activity for a woman of her stature.

In 1847, at age 27, she was sent on a European trip with her family friends, Selina and Charles Bracebridge. It was on this trip that she met Sidney and Liz Herbert who accompanied her on visits to hospitals and convents. Sidney later became the Secretary at War in the British War Office. On the way home in 1850 she visited Kaiserwerth Institute, Dusseldorf, Germany, a hospital, infant school, orphanage, penitentiary, and training school for teachers. She stayed for 2 weeks as an observer and then returned a year later for a month for rudimentary nurse training with the deaconesses.

After Kaiserwerth, Florence Nightingale went to Paris to spend time with the Sisters of St Paul De Vincent. The Roman Catholic community had received great reputation for its hospitals, orphanages, and foundling institutions. She was determined to gain as much information and practical experience as possible to be the best nurse she could be.

On her return to England, she went to Lea Hurst. It was there that she was contacted by Liz Herbert in April 1853, as a suitable opening as a superintendent at the Institute for the Care of Sick Gentlewomen in Distressed Circumstances had been announced. It was to be reorganised and moved from Chandos Street to Harley Street, London. When the news was broken to her family, her sister wept, raged, worked herself into a frenzy, and put herself to bed.

Florence was not what the committee of the Institution expected. She gave devotion generously and did much practical nursing. She was appalled at the dirtiness of the hospital including the bed and table linens. She was determined to clean up the institute, organise the accounts, and recruit appropriate staff. Within 6 months her fame was trumpeted throughout London. In the spring of 1854, she began to visit hospitals and collect facts to establish a case for reforming hospital conditions for nurses. She started to send her data to Sidney Herbert so that he could start to bring the state of nursing to public attention. Although a better type of nurse was needed, there were none trained, and it was evident a nurse training programme was required. In the summer of 1854, cholera broke out in London around the undrained slums of the city. The hospitals were overcrowded, and many nurses died or ran away. In August, Florence volunteered at the Middlesex Hospital to 'superintend the nursing of the cholera patients'.

The summer of 1854 marked the end of the Harley Street chapter, and the apprenticeship was over. Outside of Harley Street, a catastrophe was taking place. In March, England and France had declared war on Russia, and in September the Allied armies arrived in Crimea. Florence's nursing leadership journey was about to start. She left Harley Street on 21 October 1854 with 38 personally selected nurses who were required to have had some experience nursing the sick. They arrived in Scutari, Constantinople, Turkey, on 4 November 1854. Florence was accompanied by Selina and Charles Bracebridge.

REFLECTIVE LEARNING EXERCISE

Make a list of why you entered nursing and describe your journey.
Who were your key role models and why?
Who have you influenced to make an impact on nursing?

Florence's Lifetime Achievements

This section will describe Florence's lifetime achievements from her work in Crimea until her death in 1910. Much of her work will be well known to readers of this book, but it is worth reiterating some of her outstanding contributions to nursing and society.

She was, first, a nurse. Although she was a great leader, she found no task too humble or menial, no task too strenuous or difficult, no task too lofty or remote. She dealt with everything from lice and laundry to the British War Office with the same calm efficiency that put the welfare of the sick before all other considerations.

When Florence arrived in Scutari, the day of the Battle of Inkerman, her home for the next 21 months was the Barrack Hospital. It was immense, and the sick and wounded soldiers lined the corridors. Overcrowding was accompanied by neglect, mismanagement, dirt, and disease. In a letter donated to the Florence Nightingale Foundation in 2021 by the relatives of Dr William Cruickshank, the Ratcliffe family, she wrote on 29 December to Her Majesty's Commission of Enquiry (Fig. 1.1). This letter demonstrates her determination to speak to authority, to reduce the appalling conditions and the death rate, and reform conditions.

Following Florence's return from Crimea in 1856, so great was the public's admiration for her work that a public fundraising appeal was launched and over £44,000 was raised. This became the Nightingale Fund. The fund was used to build the Nightingale Training School at St Thomas's Hospital, London. The Fund still exists today.

FLORENCE'S NURSING LEADERSHIP ATTRIBUTES

The reader can reflect on Florence's leadership attributes and those attributes needed by nursing and midwifery leaders today.

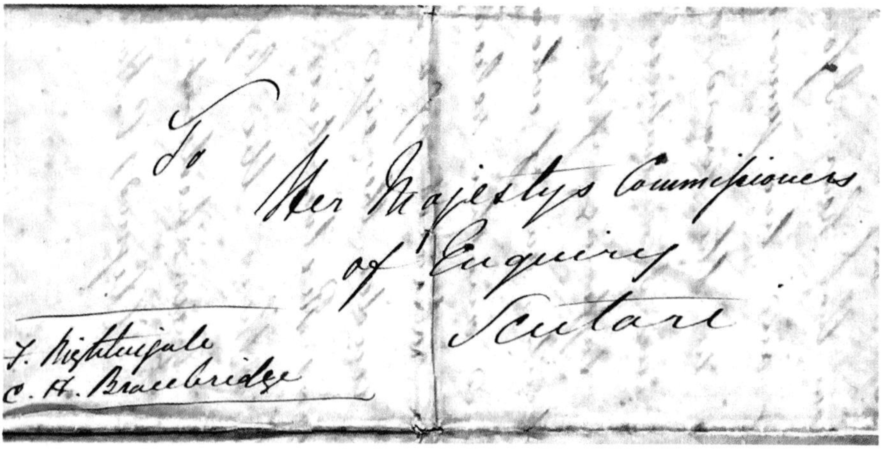
To Her Majesty's Commissioners of Enquiry Scutari

F. Nightingale
C. H. Bracebridge

Figure 1.1 Nightingale's Letter to the Commission of Enquiry.

29 Decr 12.30 A.m.

Gentlemen

I have the honor to inform you that at 8.30 last night I visited ward 17 in corridor C where I found 43 patients about 20 of whom were wounded. I was informed by the Orderlies that these had had tea and bread from the Stores as well as wine, also arrowroot from my kitchen. the ward was devoid of utensils and the men on the ground (the boards and trestles were in the next ward) I was told three Med. men had been there. Mrs Roberts and I began to make the men comfortable and I sent for hot water and water bottles &c. As no Medical men returned by 10 I went in search of the Orderly Officer for the night but not knowing where to find him I called out Dr McGregor from his quarters

Figure 1.1 cont'd

I was led to this irregular act
by finding the mens wounds un=
-dressed, many very ill, and one
man expiring, who died before 10
P.m. On the arrival of Dr McGregor
he summoned the Orderly Officers
(whom we met) and the patients
were dressed & attended to till 14.10
this morning. During this time war
&c. was administered and hot water
applied. One man died at midnight
and one ball was extracted by
Dr McGregor from the face of
another. When I and my nurses
retired several others of the sick
patients were in a most dangerous
state. I presume that the urgency
of the case may excuse my
irregular application to Dr McGregor
for which I intend to apologise
to the Medical Officer of the
Division and I have the honor to be

Gentlemen

Your obedient servant

Florence Nightingale

Figure 1.1 cont'd

Identifying a Problem and the Solution

Florence was not only a 'sick' nurse but the organiser of hospitals, organiser of professional training for nurses, and a 'health' nurse. She identified the need for 'district' nursing in 1876. Florence introduced trained nurses in the workhouse infirmaries in Liverpool. She laid the foundation of public health nursing. She attacked puerperal fever in lying-in hospitals by collecting facts, and she drew conclusions in light of statistical evidence. In 1876 she lobbied the government for a midwifery training programme. In 1902, the first Midwives Act was passed.

She was a forerunner of the doctrine of prevention rather than cure and saw education as the best means of prevention. She envisaged the district nurse as the teacher of health. Nightingale's plan for military nursing was implemented during the First World War in 1914.

Even this was not enough. She attacked the problems of lack of services in Crimea and public health in India, and she was far ahead of her time in using graphs and charts to illustrate her findings.

Influencing With Authority

Florence Nightingale was also adept at what we now call social influencing, as she wrote and received thousands of letters, reports, and books, influencing reform in many areas. This was mostly achieved after she returned from Crimea until her death in 1910. Florence Nightingale, through her writings and networks, was a health promotor and public health activist.

Florence used **social networks** to influence her work. As a Victorian woman she did not have a voice, but she convinced Sidney Herbert in Parliament to raise her issues and to be her voice. It is imperative as nursing and midwifery leaders that we use our authority to reform our work.

Using Data

Florence achieved so much reform using data. Florence was a researcher and statistician who worked with the leading statisticians of her time. She knew the importance of collecting and analysing data, presenting it in a form that people could understand, and most importantly using the findings to influence political and social change. With the statistician Dr William Farr, she developed ways to present data on deaths in Crimea in a visual format and compared this to the number of preventable deaths from infections during that conflict (Fig. 1.2). Today we use digital data, and it is incumbent upon us to use data to change practice and become nurse and midwife digital leaders.

Using Passion to Tell the Story

Florence Nightingale was a thinker and philosopher, seeking understanding of the complex universe and the ways of God. She used her passion to influence nursing and contributions to public health worldwide, and indirectly through the emancipation of women and her assistance to India, the Army, and the workhouse. She had incredible presence and frequently had audiences with Queen Victoria and Prince Albert. Her passion to change the health of the nation captivated them.

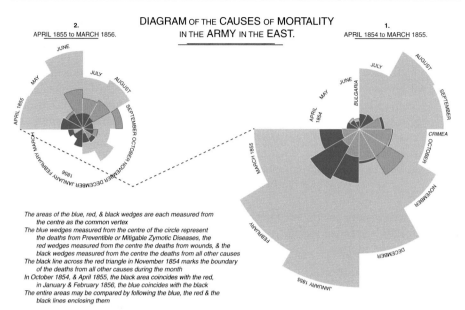

Figure 1.2 Florence Nightingale's diagram illustrating the causes of mortality of the British Army in the Crimean War, 1854 to 1856.

REFLECTIVE LEARNING EXERCISE

Make a list of your nursing achievements and the impact you have made.

What was your greatest achievement and why?

What would you still like to achieve?

What is your plan (timeline, nursing/midwifery roles needed, people to work alongside) to achieve this vision? Write your plan.

Florence's Significance and Relevance Today

This section will align Florence Nightingale's work and its significance to the global COVID-19 pandemic. In March 2020, Florence Nightingale's bicentenary year, the world locked down to battle the COVID-19 pandemic. At the time of this writing, restrictions are still in place across the world to prevent the further spread of new variants of the virus. Nurses and midwives across the world have been on the front line from the start. Sadly, equal numbers of nurses and midwives across the world have died during the COVID-19 pandemic than during the First World War (Catton, 2020).

Florence's awareness that the environment has an effect on the spread of disease is evident from her data analysis of the mortality rate in the Crimean War (see Fig. 1.2). Florence had implemented hand washing and other hygiene practices in British army hospitals.

Like many public health experts of her age, Florence considered the home to be a crucial site for disease-preventing interventions. This was the place where most people contracted and suffered from infectious diseases. This is true today in the transmission of COVID-19. Later her observations and conclusions are documented in Notes on Nursing (1860) 'True nursing ignores infection, except to prevent it' (p. 20). 'Every nurse ought to be careful to wash her hands very frequently during the day. If her face too, so much the better' (p. 53). The book was more of a public health instruction book than a nursing manual. It advised ordinary people how to maintain healthy homes. Florence strongly advised that people open windows to maximise light and ventilation and displace 'stagnant, musty and corrupt' air. She advocated improving drainage to combat water-borne diseases like cholera and typhoid.

REFLECTIVE LEARNING EXERCISE

Describe your role during this pandemic.
Imagine nurses and midwives reading this account in 100 years. What would you like them to know as a historical account?

The Florence Nightingale Foundation Today, Florence's Legacy

The story of the Florence Nightingale Foundation (FNF) is linked with the early history of the International Council of Nurses and the Florence Nightingale International Foundation. This section describes the origins of the idea for a memorial to Florence Nightingale, proposed to the International Council of Nurses (ICN) in 1912, the formation of the Florence Nightingale International Foundation (FNIF) in 1934, and later the establishment of national Florence Nightingale memorial committees. The original FNIF scholarships were undertaken in collaboration with Bedford College, and scholars were housed at 15 Manchester Square, London, during their scholarship year. Operations were cancelled during the Second World War. The current FNF derives from the Florence Nightingale Memorial Committee of Great Britain, contributing to almost 110 years of Florence Nightingale memorial history.

1910–1913

Following the death of Florence Nightingale in 1910, the international nursing community wished to pay tribute to her life and work. At the 1912 ICN Congress in Cologne, Ethel Bedford Fenwick, the ICN's first president, in her speech at the final banquet, proposed that 'an appropriate memorial to Florence Nightingale be instituted'. She envisaged an educational foundation which would enable nurses 'to prepare themselves most fitly to follow in her footsteps'. It was enthusiastically endorsed by the delegates. A committee was set up to explore ways and means but World War I intervened before any action could be taken.

1914–1934

The First World War brought nurses to the forefront of the public mind. The necessity for an immediate trained group of nurses to assist the devastated countries of Europe led the League of Red Cross Societies to offer a series of approximately 20 annual scholarships for nurses from all countries to be held in London for 1 year. They formed part of the Public Health Courses offered jointly by the College of Nursing and Bedford College (University of London). These courses came to be known as 'International

Courses'. In 1924 the League leased a house at 15 Manchester Square, London, where the students lived together during their year in London. The students who completed these courses formed the 'Old Internationals' Association' and were known as 'Old Internationals'.

The Florence Nightingale Memorial proposal was finally activated at the 1929 ICN Grand Council in Montreal. Ethel Bedford Fenwick was elected Chairman of the Florence Nightingale Memorial Committee. The question of an autonomous foundation sponsored jointly by the ICN and the League of Red Cross Societies taking over the International Courses and 15 Manchester Square was debated in many parts of the world. By 1930 the League had difficulty in financing the International Courses but was of the opinion the courses had served their purpose in creating a body of nurses prepared to give leadership in the nursing world, and especially in war-torn Europe. The League could no longer justify the expenditure of vast sums for this purpose, but 216 students from 41 countries attended these courses between 1920 and 1933.

The International Courses were seen by some as a possible nucleus for such a memorial. Professor Adelaide Nutting, a Canadian born and American retired nurse, stated 'Florence Nightingale belongs not alone to England and the English people. She is one of those whose home is the Universe. Her work is the work of all humanity'. In a letter dated 3 July 1929 to Nina Gage, president of the ICN, Adelaide Nutting wrote, 'In keeping with this new conception of a memorial as something beyond a shrine – something filled with a living, growing purpose – is the idea which I believe we should try and embody in a Florence Nightingale Foundation. It should not be restricted to the achievement of a single object, but devoted to the development of educational work, instigating and assisting important lines of research in the fields of Miss Nightingale's greatest interest, the publication of studies, reports and monographs – there are many yet to be written about various phases of Miss Nightingale's own work: to the creation of certain fellowships for students of unusual promise, and to such other activities as the years may show the necessity for undertaking.

The Foundation should be created through the initiative of the International Council of Nurses with the active cooperation and support of individuals and societies of suitable character. It should be established in the form of a permanent Trust, endowed and under the direction of a body of Trustees composed of men and women of very great eminence, representing different countries, and including, if possible, some member of Miss Nightingale's family'.

The Florence Nightingale Memorial Committee, at an ICN meeting in 1931, proposed for the memorial to take the form of a foundation for the postgraduate education of nurses. It was also proposed that individual national Florence Nightingale memorial committees should be set up in the countries of ICN member associations.

On 5 July 1934, the FNIF was established and became an autonomous organisation under British law with its own governing body. The Trustees were the Westminster Bank Trustee Department (London). Twenty-one national Florence Nightingale memorial committees were also established within ICN member organisations.

The objectives of the FNIF were stated in the Trust Deed as:

1. To establish and maintain a permanent International Memorial to Florence Nightingale in the form of an endowed trust for postgraduate nursing education either in continuation of the postgraduate courses for Nurses hitherto organised

by The League of Red Cross Societies and conducted in conjunction with the College of Nursing by Bedford College for Women (University of London) or otherwise.

2. The maintenance and development of facilities for postgraduate education for selected nurses from all countries.

1935–1945

The Second World War finally decided the fate of the courses. The 1939–1940 course was planned, and students had started to arrive, but by the end of August war was obviously imminent and the students were hastily repatriated. Manchester Square had been destroyed in an air raid during the war in September 1940.

1946–1955

The war years had affected the British national committee, and it wasn't until March 1946 that the Florence Nightingale Memorial Committee (FNMC) of Great Britain met for the first time since 1939. In 1947 the Duchess of Marlborough was elected as chair and reconstituted the National Florence Nightingale Memorial Committee of Great Britain and Northern Ireland.

At the same time, in September 1946, the Grand Council of the FNIF resolved that 'the Grand Council, having considered the recommendation presented to it by the Board of Directors of the International Council of Nurses, agrees that the FNIF make a Study of its organisation, function, procedure and programme. Inasmuch as the International Council of Nurses expects to conduct a similar study of its own organisation, the Grand Council agrees that those responsible for these two studies confer jointly before final action is taken by either body'. Each committee reported back to its own governing body with recommendations, the main one being that FNIF should be associated with or function within ICN as a legal entity and retain its own trust, deed, and funds. Both organisations agreed, and a joint planning committee worked on the details with the expectation of agreement and handing FNIF over to the ICN.

An immediate and urgent task was to find a replacement for 15 Manchester Square. A new FNIF headquarters was established at 45 Gloucester Place in 1945, with the decision not to revive the International Courses but to develop new educational policies. As an interim policy, FNIF arranged studies for selected nurses who had approached the Foundation through their national committee, or where one did not exist in a country, through the National Nurse's Association or national Red Cross Society. The Foundation arranged opportunities in postgraduate schools or universities or attached students to schools of nursing or other relevant institutes.

The FNMC of Great Britain committee opened Burleigh House, 173 to 175 Cromwell Road, London, in September 1948 in time for the new academic year, and with the permission of the Nightingale family the name was changed to Florence Nightingale House. It is by this name that it is still remembered. The residence accommodated 40 people. Some furnishings salvaged from 15 Manchester Street were donated and used to decorate eight bed-sitting rooms.

In 1951 a new member was appointed to both the committee and the council, Mrs Kathleen Dampier-Bennett. Her contribution was to open a new line of activity for the committee, for she brought its work to the attention of her son, Major (later Sir) Dan Mason. He also joined the committee, and they interested a family trust to fund the committee for nursing research.

The incorporation of the National Florence Nightingale Memorial Committee of Great Britain and Northern Ireland took place in April 1953. FNIF asked that all scholarships awarded by national committees followed policies drawn up by FNIF, and this was agreed. The Foundation also requested that the scholarships be named Florence Nightingale Scholarships, omitting the word *memorial* from scholarships and the title of the national committees. The British committee could not agree as the certificate of incorporation was named The National Florence Nightingale Memorial Committee of Great Britain and Northern Ireland, and this title had to be retained in the title of its scholarships and committees. FNIF also wanted all correspondence to go through the ICN member associations in each country. At that time, the National Council of Nurses, which later amalgamated with the Royal College of Nursing (RCN), requested to have copies of all correspondence sent to the ICN member associations. However, the British Committee decided to continue to correspond directly with FNIF. Finance was another source of disagreement.

The Dan Mason Nursing Research Committee first met as a subcommittee in 1954. The role of research in nursing was not appreciated at this time. Major Mason stated, 'We were starting something which nobody had ever done before, and my feeling is that we have blazed a trail along which others are now following with greater financial resources than we could ever hope for'. It was a unique and very productive period for the National Florence Nightingale Memorial Committee.

1956–1975

In 1957 the Committee was delighted when Her Royal Highness Princess Alexandra agreed to became patron of the Committee.

The first Florence Nightingale memorial service was held at All Souls, Langham Place, London. This was the first time a lamp was used in the service, a lamp borrowed from St Thomas's Hospital. It was carried through the church escorted by student nurses, and passed by registered nurses to the officiating clergy, who placed it on the altar to burn throughout the service to represent 'the undying spirit of service displayed by Florence Nightingale' and shown by nurses today.

In 1965 the service was transferred to Westminster Abbey, attended by Her Royal Highness Princess Alexandra. A Roll of Honour containing the names of all commonwealth nurses and midwives who lost their lives on active service in the Second World War, compiled by the British Commonwealth Nurses' War Memorial Fund, was introduced into the service. It is kept in the Nurses Memorial Chapel, Westminster Abbey. The Roll of Honour is carried through the Abbey by an other rank (OR) and escorted by the matrons-in-chief of the Armed Forces. The lamp is now kept on a secure shelf in the Florence Nightingale and Nurses' Chapel.

In 1965, Florence Nightingale House was closed for the work to be carried out. Students had to be relocated in hotels, and the extra cost had to be borne by the National Florence Nightingale Memorial Committee, but an upgraded building was reopened in April 1966. Her Royal Highness Princess Alexandra attended the opening party. New fees were set, but the renovation had completely drained all existing funds. Florence

Nightingale House was viewed as more valuable to the profession than were scholarships and that the money set aside for scholarships would be better spent on the house.

In 1970 the committee purchased its own lamp to be used for the Florence Nightingale memorial service with a legacy in memory of Mrs Kathleen Dampier-Bennett, a committee member from 1951 to 1968. The lamp is inscribed in her memory and was dedicated by the Dean of Westminster at the service on 12 May 1970, the 150th anniversary of Florence Nightingale's birth. It has been used at every service since.

In 1973, Lord Remnant, the treasurer, prepared a paper which posed the vital question, 'Is there a need for Florence Nightingale House?'. If the answer was yes, then the National Florence Nightingale Memorial Committee should accept a change in the aims of the charity, to allow finance to be directed more to the provision of hostel accommodation and less to scholarships. In 1975, men were accepted as residents for the first time.

1976–2017

By the mid-1970s, nurses were paid more realistic salaries and looked for a different and more independent type of accommodation, and better library facilities existed at the RCN and Marylebone Library. A formal decision was taken that Florence Nightingale House had fulfilled its purpose and should be closed. This occured in 1978. The Joint Committee agreed to give money for annual scholarships in recognition of the work of nurses of two world wars. Today's scholars may not know of the existence of Florence Nightingale House, but it not only represented 'home from home', especially to overseas nurses, but it enabled studies, usually at the RCN, at a time when salaries were low and secondment on salary from a hospital authority was a rare occurrence.

In 1994 the name of the National Florence Nightingale Memorial Committee was changed to the Florence Nightingale Foundation (FNF).

In 1995 the Foundation awarded Florence Nightingale Fellows from among its scholars who had made a distinguished contribution to the field of health care. The first fellows received their certificates and insignia from Her Royal Highness Princess Alexandra at a party following the Abbey service in May 1995. This was the first event of a national nurses' week in celebration of nursing arranged by the FNF, with widespread support from the nursing profession. The week closed with a reception at the Mansion House when several nurses were honoured for their clinical innovations in the presence of many eminent guests.

In 2013 the first of ten clinical professors were awarded the Florence Nightingale Clinical Professor title.

2018–2020

The year 2018 marked the 70th anniversary of the NHS, and to celebrate those who came from the Caribbean to build the NHS a leadership programme, Windrush was created for 70 early career nurses and midwives from an ethnic minority (EM) background. Additionally, the NHS 70 programme was established for London early career nurses and midwives. These formed the blueprint for future programmes, and since 2018, each year, over 300 nurses and midwives have completed these early career leadership programmes.

In January 2020 the Foundation launched the FNF Academy at the House of Lords at the start of the World Health Organization (WHO) designated Year of the Nurse and

Midwife. Two months later the global COVID-19 pandemic halted all FNF activities for 6 months. In September the Foundation launched membership of the FNF Academy to the Chief Nurse or the most senior nurse/midwife in healthcare organisations that employ nurses and midwives. At the time of this writing, 56 chief nurses have joined, spreading the benefits of the FNF to over 170,000 nurses and midwives in the United Kingdom.

2021

International Nurses Day on 12 May 2021 was also 201 years since Florence Nightingale's birth. The Florence Nightingale commemoration service at Westminster Abbey was the 56th, but there was no service in the 55th year as the world was locked down and nurses and midwives were called to fight the COVID-19 pandemic. The gratitude of every home throughout the world goes to nurses and midwives, who, undaunted by their own safety and uncomplaining in their constant challenges, cared for so many people during this crisis. Those who have selflessly lost their lives in the fight to save others shall never be forgotten. The socially distanced, COVID-restricted service was attended by the British Prime Minister, the Secretary of State for Health and Social care, the Shadow Health Secretary, the Minister for Care, the Chief Executive of the NHS in England, and the CNO for England, representing all UK Chief Nursing Officers (CNOs).

Helena Bonham Carter introduced her family connection to Florence Nightingale, read scripture, and quoted Florence 1872: 'For us who Nurse, our Nursing is a thing, which, unless in it we are making progress every year, every month, every week, take my word for it we are going back'. In the last year and now into 2021, the world has truly shown the progress made by nurses and midwives as they battle the pandemic.

The FNF continues to provide a living memorial of Florence Nightingale, one that would make her proud. As the current Chief Executive of the FNF, I am proud to continue her legacy through our work. I believe every nurse and midwife works hard to be their very best for the patients and the people they support. Florence was the founder of modern nursing, and of course many great nurses across the world have been celebrated since. May we all continue their legacies! May we all have the passion she had to change health and care!

Further Reading

Crawford, P., Greenwood, A., Bates, R., Memel, J., 2020. Florence Nightingale at Home, first ed. Palgrave Macmillan, Cham, Switzerland, ISBN-10:3030465330.

Dossey, B.M., 2005. Florence Nightingale's personality type: An exercise in understanding. In: Florence Nightingale Today: Healing, Leadership, Global Action. Silver Spring, MD: ANA.

Dossey, B.M, Selanders, L.C., Beck, D-M, Attewell, A., Gill, G., 2004. Nightingales: Florence and Her Family. Hodder & Stoughton, London. ISBN 10: 034082302X /ISBN 13: 9780340823026.

Hamley, H.R., Uprichard, M., 1948. A Study of the Florence Nightingale International Foundation. https://repository.royalholloway.ac.uk/file/cfbb310d-b2ba-4a67-bc5b-d3ce3e734266/1/BC_AL_335_28.pdf.

Quinn, S., 1994. The Lamp Still Burns: A Short History of the Florence Nightingale Foundation. https://florence-nightingale-foundation.org.uk/about/history-of-the-foundation/.

CHAPTER 2

Understanding Self for Effective Leadership

Greta Westwood ■ Gemma Stacey

Let whoever is in charge keep this simple question in her head (not, how can I always do this right thing myself, but) how can I provide for this right thing to be always done?
Florence Nightingale

CHAPTER OUTLINE

This chapter will explain the importance of understanding self in the discovery of a more effective leadership style. Importantly it will enable the reader to understand how leadership styles impact others and create suggestions for self-development.

The first section will explore the importance of self-awareness and emotional intelligence as core components of your leadership signature. This is your unique approach to leadership which is influenced by your values, formative experiences, and in-depth understanding of your internal motivations and desire to lead.

The second section of this chapter is illustrated through the concept of the Myers–Briggs Type Indicator (MBTI). It assumes the reader has self-completed the MBTI assessment. Understanding MBTI identifies how individuals see and interact with the world, own motivations, and understand the motivations of others. It creates a strong foundation for personal growth and development. It enables lifelong personal development, using a constructive, flexible, and liberating framework for understanding individual differences and strengths.

OBJECTIVES

- Explore the concept of a leadership signature
- Reflect on the importance of emotional intelligence and self-awareness
- Introduce the concept of the MBTI and preference pairs
- Explore leadership styles using MBTI preference pairs
- Examine Florence Nightingale's leadership style through the lens of her assumed MBTI preference
- Explore personal development needs to become a more effective leader using reflective exercises

15

Defining Your Leadership Signature

A central component of effective leadership development is a commitment to understanding how your personal values and formative experiences have shaped you and your approach to leadership. You will have encountered leaders who exude a strong sense of authenticity. This can be attributed to an alignment between their internal motivations to lead and their external leadership behaviours. You might assume this is a natural attribute which is more about the person they are than the development they have engaged in. This assumption is likely to be far from the truth. An enhanced level of authenticity requires in-depth personal reflection, a willingness to explore and learn from mistakes, and the impetus to seek feedback from others whom you lead. All of this requires the leader to be comfortable with showing vulnerability and humility.

Your personal leadership signature refers to your own unique approach to leadership which is underpinned by your values, experiences, and internal motivations. The following questions will help you to begin the process of defining your leadership signature; however, a commitment to ongoing reflection will be required.

1. What formative experiences have influenced your approach to leadership?
2. What influences your motivation to want to be a leader?
3. What do you hope to achieve through your leadership?
4. What attributes do you value in your colleagues and team members?
5. What attributes do you value in those whom you view as more senior leaders?

You may be able to answer these questions quite easily on a superficial level, however to get to the core of these questions you will need to ask yourself several times. This is known as Socratic questioning, for example:

Q: **What influences your motivation to want to be a leader?**
A: I want to make a difference to people who receive care in the service where I work and improve their experience.

Q: **What else influences your motivation to want to be a leader?**
A: I can see how practice which is routine and embedded could be improved and it frustrates me that we continue to repeat the same mistakes.

Q: **What are the implications of this?**
A: I hear from my team that they feel conflicted by the way that they want to practice and the way they can practice. I can see that we will lose them, or they will stop caring if they don't feel heard and things do not change.

Q: **What evidence do you have which supports this?**
A: I feel that I have a trusting relationship with my team, and I am coming from a strong position to make the changes that we can all see are needed. I want to have a wider influence on my service, and I can't achieve that on my own.

Within this dialogue you can start to understand the values and internal motivations this person holds. It is often only when values are challenged or restricted that it becomes clear how important they are. This can have a negative effect on a person's morale. Conversely, it can become a motivation to want to lead and create positive change.

Defining your leadership signature is a process which starts with internal reflection and can be refined through strategies which develop our self-awareness and emotional intelligence. Self-awareness refers to the conscious knowledge of your own character, feelings, motives, and desires. Integrating self-awareness into your professional development as a leader is shown to support emotional availability, self-regeneration, and increased personal and professional fulfilment even when faced with difficult and/or emotionally challenging situations (Sabo & Vachon, 2011).

Self-awareness is identified as a core component of emotional intelligence which is defined as the ability to understand and manage your own emotions as well as recognise and influence the emotions of those around you. Increasingly, high emotional intelligence is recognised as the most influential factor in successful leaders and exceeds the importance of technical knowledge or expertise. Common traits identified in leaders who have high emotional intelligence are listed below:

- An understanding of your personal strengths and weaknesses.
- A recognition of your emotions and how they affect your team.
- The maintenance of a positive outlook despite stressful situations or setbacks.
- The ability to respond calmly and considerately as opposed to being reactive to the immediate challenge.
- An awareness of the impact group dynamics play within an interaction or amongst a team.
- A motivation to understand a colleague's feelings and perspectives and adapt your communication approach accordingly.
- A commitment to influence, coach, and mentor others.
- A willingness to actively seek to address conflict within teams and have challenging conversations which call out behaviours that are destructive or unproductive.

Several practical ways can be used to enhance emotional intelligence. These include initiatives such as continuing education, peer support, mindfulness meditation, 360-degree feedback, and reflective writing. Each of these are purposeful acts which demonstrate a commitment to understanding self. This reiterates that authentic leadership is not a natural attribute or quality. It is highly likely the leaders you admire engage in purposeful activity which offers them the thinking time or feedback that contributes to their emotional intelligence.

REFLECTIVE LEARNING EXERCISE

Let's return to the question 'What attributes do you value in those whom you view as more senior leaders?' and add a supplementary task. Seek out a senior leader or peer with the attributes that you value and ask them about the strategies they utilise to develop their emotional intelligence. Gather their perspective on the value and purpose of these acts which enhance self-awareness and consider what strategies you might adopt.

Exploring your personality preferences through psychometric frameworks such as Myers–Briggs Type Indicator (MBTI) can further enhance your understanding of self. Understanding MBTI identifies how individuals see and interact with the world, their own motivations, and the motivations of others. The following section will discuss the principles of MBTI and offer insights into how this framework can enhance your emotional intelligence through an in-depth understanding of self and others. The understanding of personality preferences will further enhance the definition of your personal leadership signature, as you will see how each of us offer our unique personalities, including strengths and blind spots, to our leadership practice.

Myers–Briggs Type Indicator (MBTI)

The MBTI is based on Carl Jung's theory of psychological type. Jung suggested that personality can be shaped by three sets of preferences for the following:

1. Orienting oneself in the world (extrovert or introvert)
2. Collecting information (sensing or intuition)
3. Making decisions (thinking or feeling)

The MBTI questionnaire was developed in 1942 by Isabel Briggs Myers and her mother, Katharine Cook Briggs. They added a fourth preference: the way in which one lives one's life (judging or perceiving).

1. Where you focus your attention – extraversion (E) or introversion (I)
2. The way you take in information – sensing (S) or intuition (N)
3. How you make decisions – thinking (T) or feeling (F)
4. How you deal with the world – judging (J) or perceiving (P)

MBTI therefore determines that an individual will have a preference in each of the four dimensions. The four preference pairs are shown in Fig. 2.1.

An MBTI preference type is therefore made up of four letters, one from each preference pair. Understanding this preference type can help individuals explore self and interactions with others. Fig. 2.2 illustrates the preferences into 16 MBTI 'Typies'.

LEADERSHIP PREFERENCE AND IMPACT ON OTHERS

The MBTI profile reveals how we see and interact with the world, giving insight into our motivation and the motivation of others. This provides a strong foundation for personal growth and development, underpinning enhanced personal effectiveness.

The MBTI tool is often used in leadership development and provides the individual with a positive framework to explain how we interact with the world and each other using both internal and external factors to the workplace including:

- Conflict
- Resilience

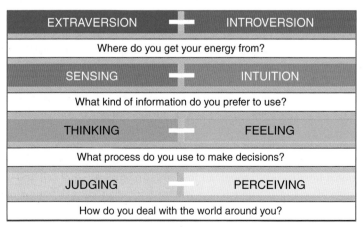

Figure 2.1 MBTI Preference Pairs.

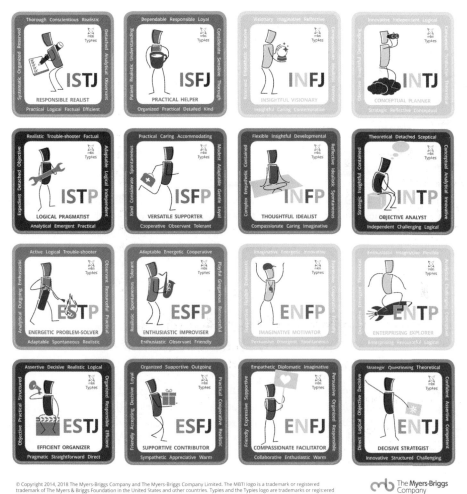

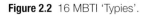

The **Myers-Briggs** Company

Figure 2.2 16 MBTI 'Typies'.

- Teamwork
- Communication
- Decision making
- Influencing
- Emotional intelligence
- Career development
- Managing others
- Managing change
- Leadership

This section will explore how each preference type has a unique way of leading.

When we think of leadership skills and personality types, we often think of the more 'domineering' types, ENTJs and ESTJs. But each personality has a unique way of leading. Some types are given more opportunities to lead than others, and other types lead 'in the background' by making suggestions and subtly manoeuvering situations to their rightful course. Understanding individual personality types through the lens of the MBTI will help you understand how to be a more effective leader and how leadership styles can impact others. Any type can be a leader, but every type is going to do it a little bit differently. *Psychology Junkie* has named each MBTI preference type as a leadership style (Storm 2017).

ISTJ – The Detail-Oriented Leader

ISTJs are quiet, careful leaders. They want to make sure that the people they lead have a clear direction; consistent, honest leadership; and a logical plan of action. They may feel an irresistible urge to organise people and take charge of projects. They will take plenty of time to make sure their plans are detailed, accurate, and fact-based. They will make it easy for everyone to understand where they're going and how to get there. When making decisions for the organisation or team, they will focus first on the facts and details, and then they will look at the pros and cons. Through everything, they will try to stay objective and fair.

Possible Struggles: ISTJs can get so caught up in the details of a problem that they lose sight of the big picture. They can also have difficulty taking into account the emotions and needs of everyone they lead. Tactfulness and empathy can be a struggle for ISTJs who aren't in touch with their feeling function. They should ask intuitive and/or feeling team members how to maintain morale and get their desired, big-picture outcomes.

ESTJ – The Decisive Leader

ESTJs are known as objective, efficient, and fair leaders. They get a thrill from making tough decisions and organising a team to get a job done quickly. They are practical, sensible, and down-to-earth. While they may seem domineering to many, they truly enjoy collaborating with people and coming up with goals as a team. When they make decisions, they will look at the facts, the pros and cons, and the most logical process. They are no-nonsense, practical leaders and will generally be quick to find a clear direction and stay with it.

Possible Struggles: ESTJs have to be careful not to 'steamroll' over other people's working styles, emotions, and differences. They may become so focused on pros and cons that they ignore how decisions might affect people in a personal way. They can also struggle with micromanaging the people they lead. They usually have a very clear idea of what they want and may have difficulty being open-minded to the suggestions of intuitive types.

ISFJ – The Thoughtful Leader

ISFJs are extremely committed, conscientious, and devoted leaders. They know how to stay organised, meet deadlines, and care for their team. They will be careful not only to make sure jobs are done well but to make sure harmony is maintained within the group. They are generous, thoughtful, detail-oriented leaders. They give specific instructions, are clear in their expectations, and will put the needs of their team above their own needs in many cases. When ISFJs make decisions, they will first consider how those decisions will impact other people. They will also look at the facts, details, and practical implications.

Possible Struggles: ISFJs are good at staying on track with goals, but they may struggle with knowing which goals to prioritise. They may struggle with seeing 'the big picture' or developing strategy effectively. They may also try to avoid confrontation to such a degree that they struggle with making decisions. If a decision might negatively impact anyone in their team they may not know how to move forward. Having one or two advisors who have a thinking or intuitive preference can help them to manage the strategic aspect of leading.

ESFJ – The Generous Leader

ESFJs are encouraging, charismatic, and hard-working leaders. They empathise greatly with people and use that empathy and compassion to ensure that everyone is taken care of and heard. They are dedicated to their team and their shared goals, and they work in a timely, efficient manner. ESFJs are often called 'servant leaders'. This is because they will put the needs of their team ahead of their own needs. If a crisis erupts, the ESFJ will be helping and supporting others instead of looking out for themselves. They are very caring and task-oriented individuals who will lead with kindness and clarity.

Possible Struggles: While ESFJs are experts of diplomacy, they can struggle with strategy and long-range planning. They are good at short-term task completion and practical planning but taking strategic risks for the long-term benefit of an organisation or team is a struggle for them. They also may struggle with remaining objective. They desire so much to maintain harmony in their group that tough decisions or prioritising the needs of the organisation or vision over keeping everyone happy can be difficult for them. If they can keep a thinking and/or intuitive type in an advisor position, this can help them to ensure they balance their need for harmony with a logic-driven process.

ISTP – The Tactical Leader

ISTPs are quiet, observant, and effective leaders. They are open-minded and casual, focusing on realistic opportunities, plans, and tactics for success. They are willing to hear many perspectives and prefer to 'live and let live'. You don't have to worry about being micromanaged by an ISTP; they like to give others the freedom to find their own unique paths towards success. They like to work alone, and they strive to find the most effective way to achieve goals using the least amount of unnecessary labour. They are adaptable, cool-headed in a crisis, and excellent at troubleshooting. When they decide, they will first think of the most logical approach. After that, they will try to find the most efficient, streamlined course of action.

Possible Struggles: ISTPs are good at solving problems in the present moment, but they can struggle with seeing a long-term vision or plan. They may also be so impersonal that they can ignore the emotional needs of others. They may struggle with being 'tied down' to an organisation, especially if they start to disagree with values. They tend to work best alone and may turn down leadership opportunities if they feel it will infringe on their space. If they are determined to be in leadership positions, they often benefit by having intuitive and/or feeling advisors who can help them to come up with a long-range vision and maintain positive morale in their group.

ESTP – The Fearless Leader

ESTPs are charismatic, effective, and fun-loving leaders. They are excellent at seeing opportunities and taking advantage of them quickly. They are skilled troubleshooters, inspiring speakers, and usually lend humour and adventure to any endeavour. They are masters of solving problems on the fly and facing adversity with courage and optimism. ESTPs will try to be as logical as possible when making decisions. They will think of the pros and cons and try to find the most streamlined, effective path towards success. ESTPs tend to know how to present plans in a way that will motivate others and maintain morale.

Possible Struggles: ESTPs are quick to see opportunities but often find the technicalities of reaching a long-range vision frustrating. They don't tend to enjoy dwelling excessively on the future and can tire of planning ahead. ESTPs also love their personal freedom and can feel trapped if they are stuck in an organisation or culture that asks too much of their time. They may struggle with staying committed to a vision or plan, always seeing new and different opportunities that seem more appealing. ESTPs who are committed to leadership can be helped by having an intuitive advisor to help them with some of the theoretical, long-range planning.

ISFP – The Sensitive Leader

ISFPs are unassuming, gentle, and compassionate leaders. They are good listeners, adaptable in their vision, and empathetic in their approach. They usually lead quietly, and will only seek out leadership positions in companies or organisations they truly believe in. They work best if they are leading a cause that will help people, especially those that are persecuted or marginalised. They believe in standing up for the underdog, so this is often where you'll see them lead most determinedly. When ISFPs make decisions, they will first consider how that decision aligns with their conscience and values, then they will think about how that decision will impact the people involved.

Possible Struggles: ISFPs tend to be flexible and hands-on in their work and can feel frustrated if they are stuck in an office all day with rigid rules and deadlines. They can feel overwhelmed by long to-do lists and by living up to the expectations of other people. They can also have difficulty finding the most logical, objective approach to meeting a goal. Delivering tough news to teammates or firing people can be extremely stressful for them. ISFPs who are determined to be in leadership would be helped by having intuitive and/or thinking advisors who can help them to see strategic, long-range plans, and can handle critiquing or correcting employees or teammates.

ESFP – The Charismatic Leader

ESFPs are extremely likeable, fun-loving, and inspiring leaders. They are in-tune with the needs of their team and will lead with honesty and compassion. They get excited about new opportunities, and they are quick to adapt to changes. They don't mind getting 'into the trenches' to get a job done and to connect with the people around them. They know how to lift up their teammates, encourage them, and make the most of each moment. When they make decisions, they will first consider how realistic or exciting the outcome will be. They will also think about how that decision will align with their values and how it will impact the people involved.

Possible Struggles: ESFPs are free spirits who don't like to be tied down or overwhelmed with long to-do lists. They can struggle with long-term commitments unless that commitment stirs their values or compassion for people. ESFPs like to take advantage of the moment, and they are excellent at solving problems spontaneously, but they can tire of focusing extensively on the future. They can also struggle to remain objective in decision making since they are so concerned about how decisions will impact people. ESFPs who are determined to be in leadership should get advice from intuitive and/or thinking friends who can help them with theoretical, big-picture planning.

INTJ – The Strategic Leader

INTJs lead with vision, rationality, and determination. They are guided by their intuition to see strategic pathways to a future goal. They have no problem directing, delegating, and putting plans into place. INTJs have a calm, focused demeanour that inspires confidence in their teammates. They develop enterprising plans, and they have a strong determination to see those plans succeed. When they make decisions, they will first consider how those decisions will play out in the future. Then they will think of the most efficient, logical course of action.

Possible Struggles: INTJs can get so caught up in their vision that they lose sight of details that may be important. They can also struggle with maintaining morale because they tend to disregard 'social niceties' or tact in favour of being objective and decisive. Because INTJs are intuitive-dominant, they may have difficulties putting their vision into words that will motivate sensing types. INTJs who are in leadership positions tend to be more balanced when they have sensing and/or feeling advisors who can help them to see important details and maintain morale with team members.

ENTJ – The Assertive Leader

ENTJs lead with confidence, strategic insight, and decisiveness. These straight-forward, ambitious leaders inspire confidence in their teammates. You can count on them to deliver on their promises and dream big. ENTJs will lead with honesty and say what they mean, although sometimes not in the most conscientious manner. However, their determination and hard work is an example that will motivate others. Their visionary outlook will inspire the people around them, and their rational logic and swift decisiveness will keep things moving at a steady pace. They may not be the most sensitive people in the room, but they're often the most driven and intensely focused. When they make decisions, they will first focus on what's logical and what will work quickly, followed by what will work most effectively in the long run.

Possible Struggles: ENTJs must work to take their teammates' feelings and needs into account. They are so determined to be objective and get things done quickly that they can steamroll over the feelings and ideas of other people. They can also be so caught up in getting things done quickly and so focused on their vision that they miss out on important details that need attending to. ENTJs work best when they have a mixed team of advisors. Fellow big-picture teammates can help flesh out the ENTJ's innovative ideas. Sensors can help them to see the details. Feeling types can help the ENTJ to maintain morale and consider people's personal needs.

INTP – The Unconventional Leader

INTPs lead with accuracy, knowledge, and open-minded curiosity. INTPs strive to be democratic leaders, taking in opinions and ensuring that everyone feels heard (even if they disagree with their opinions). INTPs are not micromanagers or dictators. They like to give their teammates the freedom to creatively find solutions to problems. They will step in quickly if they see their team or organisation headed toward danger. Their insight and strategic thinking make it easy for them to see how things will play out and how to avoid trouble. They have a strong vision for the future, and they will try to lead others casually and gradually towards that vision.

Possible Struggles: INTPs are extremely autonomous individuals and will tire of leadership positions that put them in crowded rooms and at the mercy of other people's schedules and whims. They tend to like leading in the background through suggestions and with plenty of space to think creatively. INTPs also dislike bureaucratic 'red tape' and get frustrated by dealing with details that get in the way of their overall goal.

ENTP – The Innovative Leader

ENTPs are enterprising, strategic, and competitive leaders. They have a knack for entrepreneurship, and they strive to challenge themselves and continually grow. They are intensely focused on their vision, always moving forward, always experimenting, always trying something new. ENTP leaders quickly see potential pitfalls and are skilled at troubleshooting and problem-solving in a crisis. They have a strong visionary focus and try to inspire that same vision and hopeful determination in their teammates. When ENTPs make decisions, they will focus first on how decisions could play out, what opportunities might be available, and then what the most logical course of action is.

Possible Struggles: ENTPs can get so excited about new possibilities that they leave other projects unfinished. They can struggle with procrastination or finding ways to prioritise their many visions and plans. They may unintentionally overwork their staff and teammates as they try to give priority to every single idea and possibility that comes into their mind. They can also be argumentative and overly competitive with their teammates, unintentionally offending others or steamrolling over their ideas or values. Many ENTPs find the advice of a trusted feeling partner helpful as they can offer advice about how to maintain morale and communicate praise.

INFJ – The Perceptive Leader

INFJs are passionate, insightful, and visionary leaders. They are most often found in leadership positions that have a humanitarian cause. They believe in taking care of their team, listening, and understanding where everyone is coming from. They are strategic in their vision, always looking forward to a future goal and finding innovative ways to get there. They are perfectionistic and demanding of themselves but encouraging and motivating to their team. When they make decisions, they will first consider how a decision will play out in the future, and how that decision will impact the people involved.

Possible Struggles: INFJs can be workaholics as leaders and can burn themselves out as they push themselves to an unattainable 'perfect' standard. INFJs also may struggle with presenting their vision in a clear way, with sequential steps and a straightforward course. Because INFJs keep their visions mostly internalised, they often feel flustered when trying to put that vision out into the world. This can be frustrating for them and the people they work with. INFJs also struggle with giving negative feedback or dealing with conflict situations. Conflict is anathema to the INFJ, and they may ignore negative situations or handing out criticism when it's needed. They are often helped by having a partner or advisor with a thinking preference who can help them to deal with conflict situations and maintain objectivity.

ENFJ – The Passionate Leader

ENFJs are charismatic, understanding, and motivational leaders. They believe in encouraging their team, leading by example, and making the world a better place. They are organised and goal-oriented, always keeping a clear eye on the future and motivating their team to work together to get there. They are very disciplined and focused, but also deeply concerned about taking care of their team and understanding where everyone is coming from. They are not afraid to get in the trenches with their team and work hard alongside them to make plans succeed. They use their intuition and feeling to navigate social settings with ease, making them excellent diplomats.

Possible Struggles: ENFJs hate conflict and try to be encouraging and withhold criticism as much as possible. This can cause negative situations to escalate as they put off dealing with them for too long. They may also be so focused on their personal relationships that they lose sight of a clear, objective, logical course of action. ENFJs can also be too hasty to make decisions and may need to remind themselves to take the time to reflect on decisions before moving forward.

INFP – The Sincere Leader

INFPs are passionate, caring, and empathetic leaders. They often take up leadership positions that allow them to fight for a humanitarian cause they believe in. They are very innovative in their plans and open to hearing many different viewpoints. They have excellent written communication skills and are skilled at conveying a viewpoint in a moving and compassionate manner. They are excellent listeners, encouraging leaders, and passionate in their pursuits. More than anything, the INFP leader longs to improve the world for people. When they decide, they will first consider how that decision will align with their values and morals. Afterwards, they will consider how that decision will affect the people involved.

Possible Struggles: INFPs are very accepting people who like to create an encouraging atmosphere for their team. They may struggle with dishing out criticism or dealing with conflict. Unless someone has violated one of their personal values, they may refrain from giving correction. They may also struggle with accepting criticism from their team. Leaders inevitably get criticism at some point from their teammates, and this can also be a struggle for INFPs who take criticism very personally. INFPs find a lot of deadlines and huge to-do lists overwhelming, and they may find themselves feeling trapped if they are having to rush to get everything done. INFPs can be helped by having advisors with a thinking or judging preference. The thinking types can help them to stay objective, and the judging types can help them to prioritise and manage deadlines.

ENFP – The Inspirational Leader

ENFPs lead with imagination, vision, and passion. They are resourceful individuals who find many innovative ways to make a difference in the world. They tend to have frequent brainstorming sessions with their team and enjoy giving everyone a chance to speak their mind. They are encouraging and uplifting, inspiring others with all their ideas and all the possibilities they see around them. ENFPs are not micromanagers, and they enjoy giving their team the freedom to complete tasks in their own creative ways. They don't mind sharing leadership and they are very open to a plethora of ideas and viewpoints. When making decisions, ENFPs focus first on the potential possibilities of each decision, then they think about how that decision will impact the people involved.

Possible Struggles: ENFPs may struggle with prioritising their many ideas. Some ENFPs try to give each of their ideas and ambitions equal priority and wind up over-working themselves or their team. ENFPs can also struggle with finishing projects. They may feel pulled to so many new ideas and projects that they lose interest in the projects they've already started and leave them unfinished. ENFPs may struggle with keeping track of the details of all their tasks. They may get so focused on their vision that they lose track of important facts and nuances that need attending to. Many ENFPs find that having an SJ advisor or partner helps them to prioritise, keep track of details, and follow through on important tasks.

The following case studies are from alumnae of the Florence Nightingale Foundation.

Case Study 1

DEEPSI – ISTJ

I am an introvert as I prefer to keep my thoughts to myself and tend to speak/share ideas only when prompted. I am a very good listener and often look at facts/data to make rational decisions. I invest a lot of time in planning as I am a perfectionist and like to pay attention to detail. I prefer consistency and routine and am more comfortable with jobs that have clear targets, roles, and expected outcomes. I take pride on being reliable, accountable, and loyal to relationships and organisations.

Understanding my personality type by using MBTI has helped me reflect on my disposition and preferences and how these might affect my interaction with others. I have realised that although I had a lot of talent, skills, and abilities within me, I often underrated these attributes and downplayed my strengths. The self-generated lack of confidence meant that my visibility, exposure, presence, and impact on the external world was limited. My personality type also influenced the career choices I made, and in hindsight I may have missed opportunities to grow or achieve promotions in my career.

I choose to challenge to myself by speaking up and engaging more. I hope to do this by participating more in group/collaborative activities and by sharing my insights sooner to ensure that balanced and effective communication is maintained at all times. I also choose to be adaptable and flexible by having greater personal and situational awareness and, if necessary, adjust my personality type to accommodate individual differences.

Case Study 2

LEONIE – ESTJ

I was under the impression that I was an introverted, detailed, intuitive person who preferred to be in my own space yet comfortable outside of my comfort zone and was admired as a leader.

I did not know that the MBTI profile could help me identify blind spots, which can help when choosing a career, performing a job, and also building relationships. I did not know that I prefer proven systems and procedures, and I am adept at organising projects, procedures, and people. I knew I always looked under the water line and thought about things outside the box before coming to conclusions.

I chose to change my belief that I was an introvert and accepted that I was not. I have chosen to be more assertive and accept how adept I am by owning the positive qualities I have and improving on the ones that require strengthening in order to function better within and leading teams.

> The impact is quite a positive one as I have seen some blind spots that could easily devalue me as a person. I better understand my personality type and have become more aware of how I could be perceived and how to articulate myself as a leader. Being organised, logical, efficient, decisive, and practical gave me a seal of approval.

Florence Nightingale as a Leader

Florence Nightingale has been described as a transvisionary leader. This model blends transactional leadership with transformational leadership. She was a leader who wanted to create mutual and permanent change, but due to her cultural circumstance, mutuality was prohibitive. She also had the vision to develop her own areas of interest including the nursing profession. Her tools were her intellect, her experience, and those she could influence to implement change. Even during her prolonged bouts of illness, she continued to work at home, and she was never derailed from her vison. Her need to provide enduring social change ensured her as a transvisionary leader. She used her expert knowledge as her power base. The perceived vision of the transvisionary leader is often viewed by others as not one that has previously been achieved or seems impossible to achieve. In this model Nightingale developed leaders rather than followers, which is more powerful than exclusively developing followers.

Nightingale was a visionary leader far ahead of her time. She was stubborn, logical, and always finished her projects. So what was her MBTI preference? Dossey (2005) studied hundreds of her letters and volumes of her work. From this Dossey identified her behaviours and then matched these to the 16 MBTI personality types (Dossey 2010). Dossey concluded her type was INTJ, and this helps us to understand her work and life. She was a genius innovator and analyst. Living her life in an introverted and structured world enabled her to achieve so much.

REFLECTIVE LEARNING EXERCISE

Describe your MBTI preference in 150 words.
  Make a list of all that you have identified about self from the MBTI assessment
  What was a surprise to you and why?
  What did you learn about your impact on others?
  What have you identified for your own development to become a more effective leader?
Describe your leadership style in 150 words.
  What are your main strengths?
  What are your challenges?
  What do you now need to begin to do to be a more effective leader?
  How do you work most effectively with your direct reports?
  What do you now know about your team?

References

Dossey BM. Florence Nightingale: her personality type. *Journal of Holistic Nursing*. 2010 Mar;28(1):57–67.

Dossey BM, LC Selanders, DM Beck, A Attewell. Florence Nightingale Today: Healing, Leadership, Global Action. 2005. Silver Spring, MD: ANA.

Healing. Leadership, Global Action; 2005. https://eu.themyersbriggs.com/en/tools/MBTI.

MBTI – the Myers-Briggs Type Indicator. https://eu.themyersbriggs.com/en/tools/MBTI.

Storm, S., 2017. Leadership style of every personality type. *Psychology. Junkie*. https://www.psychologyjunkie.com/2017/06/28/leadership-skills-every-myers-briggs-personality-type/.

Sabo, B.M., Vachon, M.L.S., 2011. Care of professional caregivers. Support. Onco. pp. 575–589. ISBN 9781437710151. Elsevier: Saunders. https://doi.org/10.1016/B978-1-4377-1015-1.00056-4.

CHAPTER 3

Developing Presence and Having Impact

Jonathan Guy Lewis

3.1 Developing the Confidence to Lead

How very little can be done under the spirit of fear.

CHAPTER OUTLINE

A crucial aspect of leadership development, which in many ways underpins all the others, is confidence. Without it, or without confidence in others, particularly those around you, how does anyone believe you? Follow you? Or even trust you?

And if you lose your confidence, or your confidence gets knocked down, how do you find it again?

In this chapter I'll be looking at what confidence means in order to do your job to the best of your ability, and how it is necessary for those around you to do the same.

OBJECTIVES

- Define the meaning of confidence.
- Examine what gets in the way of being confident.
- Discuss tools and strategies to become more confident.

Who Am I?

My name is Jonathan Guy Lewis. I'm an actor, writer, director, teacher, mentor, and coach. I have more than 30 years of experience working in both the creative sector and the wider world of communication – from playing the guvnor Chris Hammond in ITV's series *London's Burning*, Ian Bentley in *Coronation Street*, and Sgt Chris McCleod in *Soldier, Soldier* and performing in theatres all over the world to (somewhat ironically) working with newly promoted generals in the British Army and leaders of some of the biggest and most successful companies.

To date, I have worked with more than 500 Florence Nightingale Scholars in nearly a decade on leadership and personal development courses run by Royal Academy of Dramatic Art (RADA) Business.

Imagine you are just about to present a really important paper at a multidisciplinary team meeting. This really matters. Your team members are counting on you. You've spent weeks working on the content and worrying about delivering it. The fear of it has even woken you up in the night, in a sweat!

It's now halfway through the meeting and the spotlight turns to you.

You haven't really been able to concentrate on the meeting so far because you knew you were going to have to present your findings. Your mouth has gone dry. Your inner voice is getting louder. The chatter is really unhelpful, but you can't shut it up. As you are about to speak, out of the corner of your eye you catch the most senior person in the room glancing down at their watch. Then someone else seems to be stifling a yawn. You haven't even started! You want the ground to swallow you up. And now you think you might even be having a panic attack! What do you do next?

Does any of that sound familiar? If so, this chapter could be for you.

What Does It Mean to Be Confident?

REFLECTIVE LEARNING EXERCISE

Write down three qualities or factors that matter to you most when it comes to being confident.

Write down three things that get in your way, or stop you from being confident.

We can all get better at this elusive thing called confidence.

FLORENCE NIGHTINGALE FOUNDATION SCHOLAR

There is, of course, a strong and inevitable subjectivity to confidence. We all take or find confidence in our own unique ways, but here are some dictionary definitions of confidence that I think are worth sharing.

- 'The feeling or belief that you can do something well, or succeed at something.'
- 'The feeling or belief that one can have faith in, or rely on, someone or something.'
- 'The feeling or belief of being certain that something will happen, or that something is true.'

Confidence is a habit.

JONATHAN GUY LEWIS

Notice all the definitions draw on a feeling or belief rather than a thought.

Although knowing your 'stuff' is extremely important, remember something could happen 'in the moment' which might throw you.

Knowing stuff and being prepared can only take you so far. You only have to catch someone's eye or listen to some negative self-talk and all that confidence goes out of the window!

Deep, profound confidence doesn't just come from knowing things, it comes from a feeling of self-belief.

JONATHAN GUY LEWIS

It's important to frame confidence around feelings and our responses to 'fear', 'anxiety', 'challenge', and 'stress', not just around knowledge, expertise, experience, and a state of mind.

According to Clare Dale and Patricia Peyton in their fantastic book *Physical Intelligence*, there are more than 400 chemicals running around your body and brain at any one time. These neurotransmitters and hormones largely dictate how you think, feel, speak, and behave.

Understanding and managing your physiology will therefore enable you to develop higher levels of performance.

Four of these chemicals that I want you to remember are as follows:

Testosterone which we all have and produce in greater or lesser amounts. The chemical affects risk tolerance and confidence. Posture, breath, facing reality, and certain thought and emotional processes bring testosterone into one's system.

Cortisol is the 'fight, flight, or freeze' chemical. We need it to get going, but after a certain point we lose cognitive function and it becomes unhelpful. Therefore we need to have a way of managing this stuff.

Oxytocin helps us with relationships. It helps us create rapport and connection. It helps us when we need to be flexible and to work effectively in teams.

Dopamine is key in terms of achieving our goals. It creates the drive and focus we need to get the project over the line and get the job done. It's also about pleasure, new experiences, and reward.

We can absolutely influence the balance of these chemicals with strategic use of our minds and bodies.

CLAIRE DALE AND PATRICIA PEYTON

What Gets in the Way of Being Confident?

If you think you can, you can. If you think you can't, you can't. Either way, you're right.

HENRY FORD

Over the many years that I have spent with the nursing and midwifery community, and in our many discussions, I have encountered a number of common themes and challenges that include:

Imposter syndrome

Negative self-talk

Self-limiting beliefs

Fear of getting it wrong

Anxiety about having to go 'off script'

Not being prepared and being put on the spot

Being haunted by previous bad experiences
Lack of confidence or 'charisma'
Feeling intimidated
Not feeling valued
People talking over me
Uncomfortable being in the spotlight
Leaking frustrations and judgements; getting impatient
Feeling hurt or angry or both at the same time!
Forgetting what I was going to say next; freezing and then beating myself up
Physical signs: flushing cheeks, neck, sweaty palms, heart pounding
Talking too quickly!
Can't stop umming and erring

REFLECTIVE LEARNING EXERCISE

Put a tick next to any of these issues on the list above that you have felt or encountered in your career – or that you continue to experience right now.

Feel the fear and do it anyway.

SUSAN JEFFERS

We also discussed the fact that Florence struggled with her own feelings of failure, worthlessness, and imposter syndrome throughout most of her adult life – a regular crisis of confidence.

If you are experiencing a physical symptom of lack of confidence, there is a very good chance it has an emotional and/or mental component as well. For example, on the list above, if you ticked 'Physical signs: flushing cheeks, neck, sweaty palms, heart pounding', there is a very good chance that this is linked to (1) a lack of breathing, or holding your breath for too long, as you think and process and (2) negative self-talk, for example, 'I hate having to present. I know I'll go red!'

REFLECTIVE LEARNING EXERCISE

Put all the challenges that you ticked into three lists marked:
    Physical, emotional, and mental.
    Add your own specific communication challenges if they did not appear on the list.
    Now draw some lines connecting and linking these challenges across the different
        pots. See how many associations and chains of connectivity you can make.
    The page will probably start to resemble a spider's web!
    In my experience, the common denominator underlining all these issues and challenges that get in the way for most people in feeling and being confident is the following:
    Fear
    Fear of getting things wrong
    Fear of not being prepared
    Fear of not knowing enough
    Fear of being found out
    Fear of not being able to express oneself

Fear of judgement from others
Fear of humiliation
Fear of letting oneself down
Fear of losing face
Fear of being overbearing
Fear of being in the spotlight
Fear of not being liked
Fear of asking for help
Fear of not being good enough
Fear of being hurt
Fear of the fear
Fear of …
Fear of …
Fear of …

REFLECTIVE EXERCISE

Fill in the blanks. What are your personal and hidden fears?

Fear is irrational. You can be as prepared as you like, but something can happen, and it can throw you. It's happened to us all. The key is what you do next.

JONATHAN GUY LEWIS

I know what it feels like to go out on to a stage, to be in the spotlight, and to feel *the fear* – the bare, naked fear! The gut-wrenching fear that can paralyse or overwhelm you.

But crucially, I know how to stabilise myself when I catch *the fear,* to recover my *confidence,* and deliver results when it counts. Even now, to the outside world, it can occasionally look like I'm being very confident. But actually, to let you in on my secret, sometimes it is still an act. Inside, I'm still struggling. Appearances can be deceptive.

Doing my one man show *I Found My Horn* around the world and holding audiences of up to a thousand people for 75 minutes, and then playing a Mozart horn concerto at the end of it has sometimes taken me over the edge and back!

But in order to stabilise myself, I have developed some practical tools that I use every day. I teach these skills around the world and to people in all walks of life. But to reiterate, they are *my* solutions, rituals, and scaffolding, however you want to frame it, based on my own personal and anecdotal experiences. They work for me, and they seem to work for the countless numbers of people who I have shared them with over the years.

Fear is irrational.

Fear is also a habit.

So, it's useful to understand where this fear comes from.

REFLECTIVE EXERCISE

Write a few sentences by each of your specific fears about why you think you feel this fear and where it may originate.

If you don't consciously know, then spend some time, without any judgement, trying to unlock why the unconscious is pulling or pushing you towards self-sabotage.

Now write a few sentences on how you can do something positive and specific to help you let go of this fear – not control it, but let it go. Remember the more you try to control things, such as nerves, the more rigid and brittle you become.

Ask yourself questions such as:

How rational is it to feel this fear?

What are the likely outcomes of me giving in to this fear?

How proportionate is my response to the situation?

But also, please be kind to yourself. It's okay to feel these things. Let yourself off the hook. That's a good place to start from.

Another way of describing this fear could be called imposter syndrome.

This is an unwarranted sense of insecurity, and pervasive feelings of fraudulence. It was first studied by psychologist Pauline Rose Clance in her work as a therapist. Her book *The Imposter Phenomenon* was originally published in 1986. She noticed that many of her students shared a concern: though they had high grades, they didn't believe they deserved their places at the university. Some even believed that they were given their places in error. And while Clance knew these fears were unfounded, she too remembered feeling exactly the same way as a student.

It is a universal, all-pervasive phenomenon. It crosses gender, race, age, generations, and occupations. To call it a syndrome downplays how universal it really is. It is not a disease or an abnormality, and it isn't tied to depression, anxiety, or self-esteem.

Why can't so many of us shake off these negative feelings? Why do we feel that our ideas and skills aren't worthy of attention and merit? Where do these feelings originate?

We all tend to think that others are not just as skilled as ourselves, but even more so!

We can convince ourselves that they are more deserving, more talented, more anything. This can spiral into feelings that we don't deserve the accolades and opportunities over others. There's often no threshold of achievements that puts these feelings to rest.

Albert Einstein described himself as an 'involuntary swindler' whose work didn't deserve as much attention as it received.

Even after writing 11 books and receiving countless awards, Maya Angelou couldn't escape the nagging doubt that she hadn't really earned her accomplishments.

Everyone is susceptible to a phenomenon known as *pluralistic ignorance*. This is where we each doubt ourselves privately and believe that we are alone in thinking that way because no one else voices their doubts. Intense feelings of imposterism can then prevent us from sharing ideas and even applying for jobs that would be absolutely right for us.

Often it's the fear of the fear that stops us, rather than the thing itself.

JONATHAN GUY LEWIS

One of the best cures for imposter syndrome is to name it and own it. This requires speaking up about it and actively engaging in conversations and encouraging others to own it too. Many people are too afraid to talk about it as they fear that their fears will be confirmed. Even when they receive positive feedback, they are waiting for and expecting the negative bit as well – 'What's the catch?' It fails to ease their feelings of fraudulence, or they feel they are not being told the truth.

However, when mentors, coaches, teachers, leaders, and high-status figures of authority reveal that they are also experiencing these same feelings, it can often be a positive thing for others who look up to them – 'We're all in this together'. The same goes for peers. Even finding out that there is a name for these feelings can be a huge relief, and can then become a platform to build on.

What Are Some Tools and Strategies to Feel and Become More Confident?

Whether we are training actors or corporate CEOs, for me, the heart of the work we do at RADA Business is self-awareness. The more self-aware we are, the more adaptable, empathetic, and flexible we become. And the more adaptable, empathetic, and flexible we become, the more resilient and authentic we feel. And with that comes a sense of confidence.

It's up to us to adapt and flex our communication styles, not to assume or expect others to do it first. When we do take the initiative, it's amazing what often happens next!

Here is a checklist of elements that will help you be confident and to stop you lurching towards overconfidence and arrogance.

- Freedom from uncertainty, diffidence, or embarrassment.
- Faith in oneself and one's powers without any suggestion of conceit or arrogance.
- A heightened level of self-awareness and empathy.
- Boundaries in relationships – mutual respect. Being reliable and dependable. Being committed.
- Physically and vocally centred and stable.
- Having an 'energy of connection'.
- Positive self-talk and state of mind.
- Being 'visible'.
- Being clear.
- Active listening. Listen to understand.
- Having a purpose, vision, and emotional intention.
- Taking your time and making space – mental space between thoughts, and then communicating those thoughts, as well as a physical awareness of space and your relationship to it.
- A level of knowledge and expertise in a field or subject.
- A level of experience or familiarity. A proven track record.
- Being prepared and rehearsed.
- Commitment to follow through on decisions.
- Being curious and staying curious.
- Being in the moment through diaphragmatic breathing.

This last one is possibly the most important. It underpins everything.

At the heart of self-awareness, and therefore confidence, is a profoundly physical thing: breath.

BREATH

I bet that as soon as you read the word 'breath', you took a breath.

You've become aware of your breathing at the very least. Either holding it as you've been reading or consciously taking a breath now. And that is typical of how we function.

When we become absorbed with thoughts and thinking, we often forget to breathe – to stay connected with our 'centre', our gut, our power.

Or we get into the habit of breathing in a relatively shallow way – what's called a 'top up' breath. We survive, but this habit does not help us thrive.

It's scary to let go of shallow breathing because it's so habitual…natural…instinctive. It feels safe.
FLORENCE NIGHTINGALE FOUNDATION SCHOLAR

Deep, centred diaphragmatic breathing creates an energy of connection between us. It heightens awareness and empathy. It gives you time to think before you speak. And these breathing exercises are at the centre of many ancient practices, from meditation to yoga and martial arts. When it's done effectively and consistently, it requires conscious effort. It engages your parasympathetic nervous system, which is responsible for the body's 'rest and digest' activities. It will help you to calm down and think rationally in the face of stress. When you feel happy or joyous, your breathing will become regular, deep, and slow. As a long-term investment, it can help you sustain greater emotional wellbeing.

The more common habit of top up or shallow breathing is not conscious. It can easily create the fight, flight, or freeze states of behaviour and thinking and is often linked to panic attacks. If you feel anxious or angry, your breathing will become irregular, short, and fast. It is part of the sympathetic nervous system which regulates many of our 'fight or flight' responses.

Our breath affects almost every organ in our body.

PROFESSOR IAN ROBERTSON

The way we breathe affects the levels of carbon dioxide in our blood. The latest science suggests that breathing is more than simply an exchange of gasses. By taking conscious control of your breathing, you can change the way you think and feel. By altering how quickly and deeply you breathe, you can affect your heart rate, lower blood pressure, reduce stress levels, combat anxiety, and let go of imposter syndrome – but more on that later.

One example of this is that when you take deeper and slower breaths, it can often help with insomnia.

Two recently published studies, one by a team at Yale in the United States, and the other by the University of Arizona, explored several different techniques in managing stress reduction. The studies concluded that the breathing exercises were most effective in the immediate and long-term.

Another study with veterans from the Iraq and Afghanistan campaigns who struggled with trauma found that focusing on breathing exercises normalised or stabilised their anxiety levels very quickly. They also continued to experience the mental health benefits over a year later.

What is the link between our breathing and our emotional state?

When you are frightened, you start to breathe more rapidly. This in turn heightens the sense of fear and panic which then makes you breathe even faster. You create a vicious circle. At its extreme, it can turn into a panic attack and hyperventilation. In order to break this, you have to slow the breathing right down.

There is also evidence now which shows this deeper diaphragmatic breathing can reduce pain, as well as improve decision making.

Chronic pain is amplified by stress. Your nervous system stays on high alert and is more sensitive to pain signals. So, you will therefore be more aware of them. One way of reducing this is to practice deep, diaphragmatic breathing.

Practising deep breathing exercises can also improve your decision making. It signals relaxation as your heart rate slows. It stimulates the vagus nerve, which runs from the brainstem to the abdomen. Triggering your parasympathetic nervous system will start to calm you down. I suggest you take a moment now to listen to "Take a Breath" (Mosley 2021 - https://www.bbc.co.uk/programmes/m000wc07).

REFLECTIVE EXERCISE

The best way to take a breath, believe it or not, is to empty the body of air and then simply let go. This avoids the tensions we unwittingly create when we consciously try to take a big, deep breath, from our gut. We often pull up and create tension in the chest and shoulders. Actually, our bodies know how to breathe but we've built up unhelpful habits that get in the way of our bodies being able to do this without tension. In and out through the nose, ideally. This is your diaphragmatic breath. Repeat this. Try to avoid any mouth breathing where possible. It's really not good for your body to mouth breath. Take a breath right now as you read. A big, deep breath, from your gut. In through your nose, and out through your mouth. This is your diaphragmatic breath. Repeat this. When you inhale your heart rate speeds up. When you exhale, your heart rate slows down again.

How does that feel? Not what did you think, but how do you feel?

This time, try breathing in and holding it for a few seconds before releasing the outbreath.

Is it an unusual experience for you to breathe from your gut and to actively focus on your breathing?

Are you used to living with top up breath?

By the way, it is possible to read and breathe at the same time, and to focus on both. Try it as you continue reading now.

Imagine that your body is like a machine with cogs and pistons. The machine works effectively when the cogs and pistons are operating smoothly. This requires lubrication – oil. When there is enough oil lubricating the machine, we don't even notice the cogs and pistons turning, spinning, pushing, and driving, we simply see what it produces: the output.

We only tend to focus on the machine if it starts to go wrong and needs fixing.

Oil is the equivalent of breath for your body. When there is plenty of breath flowing freely in and out of you, it's much easier for you, and for us listening, to focus on your output: the content.

Sometimes, you just need to get out of your own way.

                                                                                    BONO

When there isn't enough oil in a machine, it will start to seize up – the cogs will start to jam. And it's the same with us. Flushing, going red, or a dry mouth are the more obvious physical examples of when there isn't enough breath or lubrication. However, there any many less obvious but equally damaging symptoms and side effects.

We can catch 'the fear'. We can cause 'the fear'. States of behaviour are catching. If you yawn, I yawn.
JONATHAN GUY LEWIS

When there isn't enough breath flowing around your system, other things can and will start to go wrong with your communication. It can quickly become a downward spiral. You may start to 'leak' your true emotional responses without meaning to.

As you try to keep the lid on your frustration, anger, hurt, or fear, you could find that you are putting up barriers without even realising, as you hold your breath or shallow breathe.

As a specific example of that leak, your eye contact with someone could easily be interpreted as 'Keep out!' or 'Keep away!'

What if you attend a meeting where you feel really cross or upset but have to keep a lid on it? And at your next meeting, a key member of your team needs your support or affirmation for an initiative. What if you are still harbouring the frustration or anger aroused during that previous meeting? Or the one before that? It's not your intention to come across as 'offish' or negative or distracted, but you can't dislodge that initial anger, or hurt, from the previous meeting. You may even think you're doing a good job hiding it, but you're not. Not really. How do you think that's going to make that key person on your team feel?

By the way, you're not going to know because they may be too scared or hurt to tell you!

And they, in turn, may sit on their upset feeling. Of course, that wasn't your intention or theirs, but it may be too late. The damage may already be done.

It quickly cascades into a catalogue of repressed distress. How might that impact patients?

When you address your breathing, 30 years of experience and feedback from countless FNF scholars has taught me that many of your other issues and challenges will also start to evaporate or fix themselves as well.

Can fear can be a good thing?

The bad news is that nerves and fear never go away. They surface from time to time, but they are not something to be avoided. In truth, I'd be more worried if you didn't get them. And you need to not beat yourself up for having them or avoid the feeling altogether. They are usually a natural reaction to something you perceive as a threat. It means you care enough for it to matter to have them in the first place. But here's the thing – and one of the secrets of your future success:

Nervous energy can be harnessed for good. The adrenalin and cortisol produced don't have to be destructive. They don't have to destabilise you. They can galvanise you. They can get you onto the stage.

The key is that they need to be directed and focused, like a laser. With self-awareness, breathing, and technique, you are much more likely to be in the moment with your communication, and therefore more effective. And therefore confident.

If in doubt, breathe out.

RON MORRIS AND LINDA HUTCHISON

When you have enough breath flowing in and out of you, there's no space for fear to destabilise you. There's no room for the critical inner voice to operate. Instead, you are able to harness the positive aspects of nervous energy and redirect it in a way that is helpful.

Realistically, this takes courage, as well as technique and practice, to form this infinitely better habit.

We practice to help us act our way into change.

JONATHAN GUY LEWIS

You have to practice confidence.

REFLECTIVE EXERCISE

Make sure you aren't holding your tummy in. Let go of everything, including any vanity.
  It may feel strange or uncomfortable. Instead of a sixpack, embrace your onepack!
    Imagine you are a balloon filling up with air. It starts in your tummy, your diaphragm, this tyre or domed-shaped muscle. It continues up through your chest and even further, up into your head and down to your feet. The whole of you is filling up with this life force.
  As you take this inbreath for a count of four, give yourself positive life-affirming, internal self-talk. Here's a list of emotive words to try:

Confidence. Presence. Ease. Warmth. Flexible. Centred. Connected. Energised.

  When you're full of breath, at your maximum intake, hold it for a count of two seconds. Neither in nor out. Be in the moment with your fuel tank full. You are supplying oxygen to your brain and body.
  Then release the breath. Imagine you are blowing it out through an invisible straw. Push it out from your gut. Or imagine you are blowing out a candle on a cake. Breath shouldn't just be escaping from you. It should be energised and last for a count of four seconds.
  You are expelling the carbon dioxide.
  This is a particularly powerful exercise to calm the nerves just before performing and delivering a presentation or communicating an important message.
  At the same time as this outbreath is happening, give yourself more positive self-talk – words associated with releasing unhelpful negative feelings and emotions. You are expelling and blowing out:

Fear. Anxiety. Panic. Tension. Stress. Worry. Negativity. Anger. Hatred. Hurt. Pain.

  When your breath fuel tank is completely empty, like you've rung out all the water from a mop, hold it again for a count of two seconds.
  The reflex action to breath in will then give you a powerful inbreath of life force, or as the Italians would say, *inspere* (inspiration).
  You are actively directing your breath in and out of your body. This breathing exercise is sometimes known as the '4-2-4' method.
  If you are feeling particularly fearful, lengthen your exhales. Let it become '4-2-6', or even '4-2-8'.

You've given your brain a little reset via the vagus nerve and reduced the levels of noradrenalin in your brain. This is important for clarity of thought and managing emotions.

You'd update the software on your computer. It's important to reboot you once in a while.
                                                                    JONATHAN GUY LEWIS

Allow yourself the mental, emotional, and physical space to regularly practise this breathing exercise each day. It's something you can practise right now, at your desk, as you walk to meetings, as you pause between emails, before phone calls, anywhere and any time. You may be surprised at how quickly you feel the benefits. It doesn't take any preparation.

So much of our communication in our busy lives and busy jobs is either hampered by being in the past or in the future. By that I mean we are not totally present and in the moment.

Confidence comes from being in the moment.

But some part of us is in the habit of judging what happened, or didn't happen, or is worrying about what might or might not happen in the future.

We can carry these anxieties and frustrations from the last meeting into the next one if we don't take a moment to 'reboot' before our next encounter.

And be sure you check out your listening or concentrating face. Take a moment to check that it does not unwittingly convey judgement. I speak from bitter experience. Often, as we listen and process content, particularly difficult content, we can have a furrowed brow, or a scowl. This can be very off-putting to someone, as they may well interpret your facial expressions as negative or judgemental.

REFLECTIVE EXERCISE

Check right now to see what your face is doing as you read. Do you look approachable? Friendly? Or does your listening or processing face come across as unapproachable or unfriendly.

What might you do to change that?

Although it can be difficult to change old, embedded habits of a lifetime, this is one habit that is easier to start with. You may find it helpful to have your feet planted on the floor and awareness of your posture as you do the exercise, maybe even having your eyes closed as you do it. I will follow up on these added elements in the next chapter, Pillars of Presence.

Summary

This chapter has explored:
- What confidence actually means in a practical day-to-day sense.
- What confidence actually requires us to be doing and also not doing. Without it there is ambiguity in our communication and a potential lack of trust.
- We can think our way into being confident, but a more profound and deeper sense of confidence may come from feeling it rather than knowing it. But because we

aren't machines or robots – we feel as well as think – we have to be able to do both, at the same time.

■ Factors that get in our way – whether they reveal themselves as physical, emotional, or mental – are mostly driven by expressions of fear, and fear is irrational.

■ Imposter syndrome affects the vast majority of us at some point in our lives.

■ The main remedy to becoming confident is acquiring the better habit of diaphragmatic breathing. Conscious breathing can radically change the way you think and feel. It can improve decision making, alertness, posture, and self-talk. It drops the heart rate and helps with fears and anxieties. You just feel better.

■ It provides a physical as well as mental reset.

■ It's difficult to do under pressure, which is why it takes practise to become a better habit.

Further Reading

BBC Sounds BBC Radio 4 - Just One Thing - with Michael Mosley, Take A Breath. https://www.bbc.co.uk/programmes/m000wc07

Dale C, Peyton P. *Physical intelligence*: Simon & Shuster, London: UK; 2019.

De Cintra S. *Unlock Your Business Voice: how to speak as well as you think*. Rethink Press; 2018.

Just One Thing, With Michael Mosley, Ep: 'Take A Breath' https://www.bbc.co.uk/programmes/m000wc07?msclkid=39f07507b0be11ec87513970cb8a5358.

On managing stress (Prof Ian Robertson on managing stress - Bing video) Youtube.

Peters S. *The chimp paradox: The mind management program to help you achieve success, confidence, and happiness*. TarcherPerigee; 2013.

Robertson I. *How Confidence Works: The new science of self-belief, why some people learn it, and others don't*. Bantam Press, London: UK; 2021.

Rodenburg P. *Presence: How to use positive energy for success in every situation*. Penguin: UK; 2009.

Walter C, Brown B. Daring greatly: How the courage to be vulnerable transforms the way we live, love, parent, and lead. *International Journal of Social Pedagogy*. 2015;5(1):180–183.

3.2 Stepping Into Your Authority: Pillars of Presence

Rather, ten times, die in the surf, heralding the way to a new world, than stand idly on the shore.

CHAPTER OUTLINE

You are in the spotlight as a leader, whether you like it or not. How do you become better equipped to deal with the performance aspect of communication and leadership?

In this chapter I'll be addressing the challenges of 'walking the talk'. I'll be offering some techniques and giving you specific tips so that you can more consistently operate as the optimum version of you.

OBJECTIVES

- Clarify what is meant by my *pillars of presence*.
- Explore and address some of the barriers that get in the way.
- Identify specific and simple exercises to practice in order to create more presence.

Imagine you've just presented an exciting but controversial idea at a multidisciplinary team meeting. This is your baby. You need to sell the idea as you know it could potentially save lives and money. You need to get everyone at the meeting on board. The presentation sparks a lot of interest, both positive and negative – apprehension and doubt hang in the air. You become anxious about answering difficult questions. How do you convince, persuade, excite, and reassure everyone in the room to trust you?

Does any of that sound familiar? If so, this chapter could be for you.

Technique will set you free.

ANONYMOUS

What Are My Pillars of Presence?

Body language
Voice
Listening

Space
Ground
Intent
Rehearsal
Curiosity

These are the elements that when combined create the firm foundations on which to develop your presence. They are, in effect, the scaffolding to support you at any moment.

To have presence, you must be present. In the moment. This moment. Right now. Not the moment just gone, or the moment to come.

　　　　　　　　　　　　　　　　　　　　　　　　　　　　　JONATHAN GUY LEWIS

In our heads, we are either in the past – worrying about what happened or didn't happen – or in the future, worrying about what might or might not happen! Stay present. Be in the moment.

The people you are hoping to influence will be subliminally evaluating your credibility, confidence, empathy, and trustworthiness, and their evaluation will only be partially determined by what you say. Your use of space, physical gestures, posture, facial expressions, and eye contact can enhance, weaken, support, or crucially sabotage your impact.

BODY LANGUAGE

There is a lot of research and anecdotal material about how important body language is in the way we communicate and the effect we have on other people, as well as ourselves.

Perhaps the most ubiquitous is the famous Mehrabian study where Albert Mehrabian, now the emeritus professor of psychology at University of California Los Angeles, makes the links between body language, liking someone, and trust. (Mehrabian and Ferris 1967)

It started an entire cottage industry of experts analysing every move that we make – especially politicians and sales professionals. 'Smile while you dial' has become a massive area now. Often consultants are brought onto TV and radio shows to analyse the speakers' body language after debates and diplomatic meetings between world leaders.

However, Mehrabian's study is often misrepresented. You may see in other books on personal impact and communication skills that Mehrabian is credited with saying that 93% of your communication is about the nonverbals and only 7% about the content. Or those books may state the 7% content/38% verbal/55% body language rule.

However, this isn't actually what Mehrabian said. His premise was that when you are being congruent with your communication, we are more able to focus on your content. It's only really when communication starts to go wrong that people don't trust what you're saying and first look to visual signals. Your body language and nonverbal messaging are crucial in supporting that content. After that, they go to the way you say what you're saying, and only then do they check the content part to decide whether they trust you and what you're saying. The content part *can* drop to as low as 7% in terms of trust through your messaging. It's not a given throughout that it remains that low.

My takeaway from Mehrabian is the importance of congruence – that what you say is in sync with how you say it and how you deliver a message. This is backed up by numerous studies on body language since the Mehrabian study was published. Do I believe that you are connected to what you are saying? If you are not committed and connected to what you are saying, you will be either consciously or subconsciously planting seeds of doubt, which may then motivate me to ask you questions which you might describe as difficult.

So, in this chapter, I want to share with you a few key takeaways that relate directly to my own personal experiences in performing and teaching communication skills for over 30 years.

The way we connect with other people happens most affectingly and immediately through our body language. That may sound obvious. But even on a phone call or conference call, or Zoom nowadays, it's important to remain aware of your body language. How often have I found myself hunched over, phone to ear, and trying to focus on a complex and challenging discussion? It doesn't help my thinking, I can assure you. To remedy this I like to move around, or at least sit with good posture so that I can connect to my centred, diaphragmatic breathing as I listen and interact. (See previous chapter on confidence.)

The key to understanding the body language of presence is to become consciously aware of all your behaviours as choices. Make everything you do a choice: the way you sit, the way you look at someone, being generous with your smile to connect with others.

One size does not fit all.

FRANK ZAPPA

Flexibility is key.

A positive, energised, open posture is what we are aiming for.

Positive, open posture = positive, open thinking.

There is always a communication cost when we slip into poor body language habits – for example, what might be interpreted by habitually crossing arms and/or legs?

Just because it may feel more relaxed or enable you to concentrate, doesn't mean that it will make others feel that way too. It might have the opposite effect. If I was anxious and looking for signs of approval from you, I might interpret your arm folding as boredom or you don't like what I'm saying. Maybe you don't even like me!

We are notoriously bad at interpreting body language and often tend to project negatives onto the body language of others. It may also then lead to our own defensive, closed body language, as we often copy each other.

States of behaviour are catching.

JONATHAN GUY LEWIS

With regard to using hands, a good rule of thumb is that if you are comfortable using them, there is a good chance that I'll be comfortable watching you. If I sense that you are worried about your hands, and what you are doing or not doing with them, I'll become worried for you. The more crucial aspect to your hands is whether I can see them or not. The phenomenon of 'hidden hands' creates mistrust. This is one of the nonverbal signals that is deeply ingrained in our subconscious.

Finger pointing is also something to watch. It can signal emphasising or a need to be dominant. The problem is that it can suggest a lack of empathy or regard for the other person or the rest of the people at the meeting. It can suggest a leader feels they are losing control.

We talk about being 'in flow' with body language and mirroring when we are connecting, and interested. When you see disagreement in conversations, you won't see this flow or mirroring. You might see more of these gestures like finger pointing, or physically turning away from the other person. There might be what's called micro gestures, from small shakes of the head to more obvious ones such as raising eyebrows, eye-rolling, biting of the lip, and clenching the jaw.

Body Language While Communicating on Virtual Platforms Such as Zoom or Teams

How you show up on screen in your little rectangle is crucial. We only have our faces and particularly our eyes to do all the work. We can't see the rest of the body to make these crucial decisions of whether we trust each other. Some important things to make sure you are doing or have prepared are the following:

- Make sure there is light bouncing onto your face so that I can see your eyes. If there is too much light behind you, you will be in shadow.
- Try to have your camera or webcam at eye level. If you are looking down into your screen or keyboard or right up above the top of your screen, it can create ambiguity in terms of status. On the receiving end it can feel like being talked down to, or looking up to someone more powerful. Try and meet on screen as equals.
- Make sure that your background is not far more interesting than you are. If possible, don't have a window behind you.

REFLECTIVE LEARNING EXERCISE

Engaging the Spine

Either stand up with your feet about hip's width apart and let your arms hang down by your sides or sit in a good, solid chair with your hands facing palm down on your knees.

Sit forward so that the base of your spine is not stuck against the back of the chair. In both instances your feet need to be planted flat on the floor.

To kick things off, imagine an invisible line of thread attached to the base of your spine and running through each disc and vertebrae, carrying on to the very top of your skull and beyond.

Imagine the thread being pulled up by a centimetre, then two.

Then, imagine the tip of a pencil or rigid index finger applying a small amount of pressure on your back, right between the middle of your shoulder blades. Feel it start to push your chest bone forward. Check your shoulders are down and relaxed – become aware of the space you are now taking up with your body. Whether sitting or standing, you are thinking 'up and out of your body'.

If someone now cuts this invisible thread, see what happens to your posture. See what happens to your thought process?

Notice how the nice, open, relaxed posture suddenly crumples, and with gravity you are liable to hunch. Notice the lack of space now in your tummy. It can create anxiety, fear, and limiting or judging thoughts and beliefs.

Our body language is absolutely linked to the way we think and feel.

Now allow the thread to lift you up and out of your body again to the more stable and open physical position.

Engage your diaphragmatic breathing, and try to identify and release any physical tension that you may be holding in your shoulders, hips, jaw, ankles, fingers, and neck.

Over the course of time, with the effects of stress and gravity, we start to hunch or slump in our posture, particularly over a laptop, or a screen.

It's important during the day to check in with the physical you, your machine or instrument – to check in with your spine – to do a reset. We hold on to tension all the time, in various places, without even realising it, from shoulders to hands, necks, hips, and jaws. Our bodies hold onto anxiety and stress, otherwise.

With great risk comes great reward.

THOMAS JEFFERSON

The way you connect with other people happens most affectingly and immediately through eye contact.

You have the power to welcome people, to reassure them, to excite them. Even when feeling anxious yourself, as a leader, your team needs that nurturing and reassurance. Welcome to the world of acting! You also have the power to scare them or turn them away from you.

Their needs must come before your fears. But here's the thing: the more you give out, the more comfort you will get back.

The eyes are the windows to the soul.

SHAKESPEARE

We tend to look down or away in order to find our thoughts. I call that the 'thinking space'. It's natural to do this. We all do it from time to time.

However, when you are communicating in person, and you habitually and consistently spend more time in your 'thinking space', than in 'connecting' eye contact, the consequences for other people tend to be negative. It can feel like a barrier.

Inadvertently, you may come across as uncertain, preoccupied, distracted, bored, distant, arrogant, or plain shifty!

People tend to project negative interpretations on your lack of eye contact with them, whether you like it or not.

The expert will not come across as the expert. Even if you find it uncomfortable to do this, it's an important element to get right in order to gain and reinforce trust for others, and for them to stay connected with you.

If you're natural communication style preference is more analytical than expressive, or your energy is naturally more introverted, this will never feel totally comfortable. But it's important to be able to turn up your dial on this aspect of visual communication when necessary and to know that you can do it in order to help other people feel welcomed.

How will I know the right amount of time to hold eye contact? There is no magic answer.

The key is to make your intention positive and welcoming, and to be in the moment.

This all comes with a health warning as there are also important cultural and contextual aspects to what I've shared with you, which must also be present in your thinking and understanding.

In some cultures and societies, eye contact is a particularly sensitive issue and requires a lot of care and tact around specific norms and rituals. It requires empathy and self-awareness in order to create trust. Direct eye contact or holding eye contact for too long could be considered rude or disrespectful, or plain confrontational. It can have the opposite effect to the connection you are trying to achieve.

Certain cultures, societies, or subgroups may set deferential eye contact or signals of deferential posture as their norm. If you stray from those norms then you may be regarded with mistrust. Standing tall could be misinterpreted as confrontational or arrogant. I keep coming back to the importance of self-awareness in that particular moment, and being aware of all the signals you will be receiving both verbal and nonverbal from the other person or the group.

It's also crucial to understand and navigate the specific context in which you find yourself.

We actually make up our minds very quickly about whether we like someone. Some studies suggest it takes less than 10 seconds for us to make up our minds, maybe even 7 seconds! The human brain is hardwired in this way as a survival mechanism.

People pick up on our attitude as soon as we walk into a room. So, make a conscious choice about the attitude you want to embody.

We can, for example, make snap judgements and decisions about people based on misinformation, or nothing more than ignorance of someone and their situation, history, or culture. People may not feel they are being rude or disrespectful to your cultural body language norms. So, rather than feeling hurt or snubbed, or ignored or disrespected, it's far more powerful to stay curious.

Flexibility to turn up or turn down your dial when necessary is the key.

REFLECTIVE LEARNING EXERCISE

Ask a trusted colleague, or friend, to stand opposite you and about two meters away. First, look at them with a warm sense of welcome. Say nothing for approximately 5 seconds. This all happens with your eyes. That's important. If you find this uncomfortable or too intimate, try standing a bit further back until those uncomfortable or embarrassing feelings subside.

Ask how you came across with your connection.

Genuine, warm, friendly, welcoming?

Sometimes we think we are doing more with our expressions than what is actually being received by the other person, especially if you are more of an analytical type.

Have another go, but this time really turn up your dial of welcoming, just using your eyes. Turn it up to 11! Inevitably, you will want to smile. Let it out. Enjoy the release. It'll add to your energy of connection.

Now try the exercise again, and this time just use your eye contact with your colleague to convey anger, threat, hurt, or disdain. Use your eye connection for 5 seconds to push them away. Again, ask for feedback on how your eye contact impacted them. The difference from the first version should be very marked.

You should have two very different reactions to your two different eye connections. And it should be clear just how powerful you can be just using this eye connection, and the feelings it can summon up in people.

A smile is the shortest distance between two people.

VICTOR BORGE

A true smile begins with your eyes, and it is one of the most powerful tools or assets you have. Don't save your smile for special occasions! Be generous with your smile, unless you are conveying a sad, uncomfortable, or difficult message. It pays dividends to engage your smile as much as possible. Just like a comedian practices 'spontaneity', why not practice your smile? If smiling doesn't come easy to you, why not engage the muscles in your cheeks? Practice smiling so that smiling doesn't feel unnatural. Visualise something or someone that makes you happy and makes you want to laugh.

When you smile, your brain releases tiny molecules called neuropeptides to help fight off stress. Serotonin is also released which is an antidepressant.

REFLECTIVE LEARNING EXERCISE

Get someone to film you as you deliver a brief, welcoming, upbeat message – no more than a minute. Then watch it back. How would you feel if you were on the receiving end of this message? Would you feel welcomed and valued? Then, crucially, watch the film again, this time with the sound off. Check that visually your body language is conveying an upbeat, positive energy of connection. Check that it is congruent with the content.

Why not film a second version where you up the stakes on the smiling? When you play it back, you might be surprised.

VOICE

If I can't hear you, I don't care. If I don't care, I don't trust you. Never make me work too hard to listen to you.

JONATHAN GUY LEWIS

Key ingredients for great vocal connecting and expression include:
Volume, diction, clarity, variety, and nuance.

We humans are herd animals.

ANNA LOUISE STRONG

We collect together in groups and are very affected by the norms of that particular group or herd – any organisation or group has its rules, culture, norms, and peer pressure. The family, the football team, a choir. This is particularly so in the workplace.

As a leader, if we're not feeling confident, we can sometimes leak a need to be liked – particularly when the job gets tough.

I call it:

'The make it ok for me leak'.

For example, when we have to communicate messages from above that we don't necessarily agree with or understand, it can be hard to deliver them in a way that is convincing and congruent (matching).

Sometimes, if we're seeking approval for our content, 'The make it ok for me leak' creates a questioning tone – where we turn a statement into a question.

It's known as uptalk or upspeak.

This is different from, say, the Australian accent which tends to have a natural upward inflection at the end of thoughts (or certain English dialects and for some second language speakers). Uptalk leaks a lack of confidence, not everyday cadence. It can send mixed messages to your audience.

If you regularly or habitually turn statements into questions, you could be giving away your status and power – unconsciously seeking approval. You could be creating doubt and ambiguity for the other person. You could be giving them permission to ask you the difficult question.

Another vocal expression of 'presence' can be found in the vowel sounds and consonants of words and speech patterns. It's very empowering to understand the relationship between them, as they affect us and the people listening to us differently.

To generalise and simplify: Vowel sounds (A, E, I, O, U) carry our feelings. We express and receive feelings, our emotions, instinctively through vowel sounds.

With consonants, presence comes from clarity, diction, emphasis, and volume. This allows others to process and think about what is being said, without frustration. If your audience has to work too hard to listen, they will become distracted and may well get bored or switch off.

With vowels the following applies:

If I accidentally stub my toe on a hard surface, I would instinctively shout or scream 'Ow!' It hurt, so I express pain, the feeling, through the sound of 'Ow!'

'Ow' is a vowel sound.

I do not instinctively scream 'B!' or 'D!' or 'K!' when I stub my toe. I may possibly put a consonant in front of the vowel: 'FUUUUUUU**!!' But it's mostly vowel that carries the feeling in my painful reaction.

When we are feeling anxious, under pressure, or judged, we tend to close down the amount of physical space in our mouths to make vowel sounds. (This is a long sentence, by the way. If you were speaking it out loud, you would need to prepare by taking an even bigger breath before you speak it.)

Our jaws also tend to tighten with the stresses and strains of daily life. We then stumble over words, or can become tongue-tied! With this comes a stifling of the feeling or vowel component, whether conscious or unconscious. We get into the habit of not opening our mouths enough to speak with ease. We stifle the feeling component again. The light in our eyes dims.

We shut down to protect ourselves and to conform like the good herd animals that we are. It's deeply ingrained in our survival DNA.

The sound coming out becomes flat and uninteresting. Without enough breath to sustain the thought coming out, we can start to fall off the ends of our thoughts as we deliver them, energy-wise. This only adds to the sense that we don't really 'own' what we are talking about. The soporific effect of the falling tone can start to put people to sleep! It's often used in hypnotherapy, during a progressive induction! But one thing is certain, it is likely to induce boredom.

REFLECTIVE LEARNING EXERCISE

Try speaking the last four paragraphs out loud, without really opening your mouth, arms folded, spine collapsed, or hunched.

If you can record yourself saying this, even better.

How did speaking the words make you feel?

Not much, probably. It lacked energy. It lacked a need to connect.

Listen to it back. It's probably very uninspiring.

Try speaking the same paragraphs again. This time with an energy of wanting to connect with an audience – of wanting people to listen to you. Try it as if you were excited to tell someone this knowledge. Give each word value.

Maybe raise the stakes and imagine the person listening is profoundly deaf and having to lip read. There is an imperative to open your mouth more than feels familiar, as you speak to be understood.

When you see a full stop, take a moment to breathe – take a 'thinking breath'. (^ = Breathe)

Again, record this version. Listen back to both and compare.

^ When we are feeling anxious, under pressure, feeling judged ^ whether this is actual, or perceived, ^ we tend to close down the amount of physical space in our mouths to make vowel sounds.

^ Our jaws also tend to tighten with the stresses and strains of daily life. ^ We then stumble over words, or can become tongue-tied! ^ With this comes a stifling of the feeling or vowel component, whether conscious or unconscious. ^ We get into the habit of not opening our mouths enough to speak with ease. ^ We stifle the feeling component again. ^ The light in our eyes dims.

^ We shut down to protect ourselves. ^ And to conform like the good herd animals that we are. ^ It's deeply ingrained in our survival DNA.

^ The sound coming out becomes flat and uninteresting. ^ Without enough breath to sustain the thought coming out, ^ we can start to fall off the ends of our thoughts as we deliver them, energy-wise. ^ This only adds to the sense that we don't really 'own' what we are talking about.

^ The soporific effect of the falling tone can start to put people to sleep! ^ It's often used in hypnotherapy, during a progressive induction! ^ But one thing is certain, ^ it is likely to induce boredom! ^

How did speaking those words make you feel this time?

Energised? Connected? Present?

Speak to be heard. Speak to be understood.

JONATHAN GUY LEWIS

We speak like we drive a car. The engine goes through gears, and so do we as we talk. We don't always drive in fourth or first gear. We don't always speak at a million miles a minute! Our vocal energy and our speed of delivery fluctuates as we get into our flow. But it's important to find variety in delivery and full stops at the end of thoughts. One thought happens or travels on one breath.

Thoughts are gifts that you give to people. Watch them unpack the gift.

JONATHAN GUY LEWIS

Remember: the softer you become in volume, the more room there is in your head for the negative, censoring, doubting voice to get louder and disrupt. So, if in doubt, or if you catch 'the fear', try to get louder in volume as you speak. Then there's no room for that negative voice to put you off.

REFLECTIVE LEARNING EXERCISE

Let's practice articulation. Say: 'Red leather. Yellow leather'.

Now say it three times out loud, as quickly and clearly as you can. Give yourself between 4 and 5 seconds, maximum.

If you stumbled or tripped over the words at any point, don't worry, it's very common. It is often a sign you're holding tension in your jaw. It needs a bit of a workout, along with your tongue.

Try a slow neck roll clockwise, 360-degree turn of the head, then anticlockwise.

Open your mouth and create a yawn. Do this a few times and let sound out with it. This may trigger an actual yawn. Embrace it. Try not to stifle it. Your body is naturally trying to reboot your breath with your voice. Enjoy it, and don't forget to let some noise accompany it, from the back of your throat.

Now, massage the sides of your face with the palms of your hands and your fingertips. Use the soft pads of your fingertips on your cheeks and the skin in front of your ears, like kneading some dough.

Feel where the jaw hinges to your skull. Can you feel any tightness there?

Your jaw may even click.

As you massage your cheeks, imagine you are chewing something delicious.

Use an index finger and thumb on your chin to gently pull your mouth open.

Allow your jaw to hang down, relaxed. Say 'Ah', as if stepping into a relaxing hot bath.

Now clasp your hands in front of your face. Hold them together tightly, shake them. And say 'Ah' again – this time as if a doctor wants to check the back of your throat.

Is your face relaxed as you do this? Can you keep your jaw loose? Is it still rigid?

Do another neck roll. See if the jaw is any looser, particularly as your head hangs back with your eyes looking up.

You may instinctively start yawning again. Don't stifle the yawn or the sound. Notice the magic start to happen when you do yawn and let sound out. Feel the vibration in your chest cavity. Allow your whole body to stretch and release. Allow your body to instinctively reboot your breath with your voice.

Use the tip of your tongue to clean your teeth and the inside of your mouth. Touch the tip of your nose.

Hum up and down the range and register of the whole of your voice. Lean forward as you hum and smile. When you feel a buzzing or tickling sensation around your lips open the hum into an 'Ahhh'. Feel the sound you are making happening in front of your face, rather than in your mouth or at the back of your throat.

Repeat the 'Red leather, yellow leather' exercise. You should notice it has become easier, as you've become physically and vocally more flexible.

We can often start to feel self-conscious as we do these vocal warm-ups and exercises. Remember the benefits when you do warm yourself up far outweigh the anxiety of looking foolish. I recommend singing in the shower, or in the car, or walking. Do these exercises where you know you won't be overlooked or overheard. With practise, you will start to feel more comfortable and relaxed doing them.

LISTENING

Presence = Listening to understand.

Listening does not mean waiting for a gap in the conversation so that you can then speak or download your script at someone!

Active listening requires an element of activity from the listener so that the speaker knows they are being listened to. This may seem obvious, but look all around you at the way people communicate, and how many times the person listening is in a reflective, processing state, unaware that the speaker is looking for signals and signs of agreement, affirmation, or disagreement.

Take responsibility as the listener to connect. Don't leave it all to the speaker.

Nodding to acknowledge and to listen is a powerful affirmation to the other person. It is not necessarily a nod of agreement, but it's a clear physical sign that you value what the other person is saying. It is a powerful reminder to yourself not to scowl or have that furrowed brow. But be careful not to overdo it otherwise it can come across as disingenuous, or you can become a bit of nodding dog! Or it's something you've learnt in a course!

Remember to keep an eye on your resting bitch face!

JONATHAN GUY LEWIS

SPACE

Space = room.

Room to breathe. Room to think. Room to feel. Room to speak. Room to listen.

It's imperative therefore to make space for yourself and for others. When you make space for yourself, you give permission for those around you to centre themselves and make space as well –physical space, mental space, and emotional space.

We are often cramping ourselves in terms of one or more of these. Breathing creates and encourages space in all three of these dimensions.

Remember, and I'll say it again: 'States of behaviour are catching'.

Because we tend to think quickly, we often spin many different plates in our heads. When we do speak our thoughts, it's quite easy to fall into the habit of preparing the next thought rather than finishing the thought we are delivering. This can then create the 'umm' or the 'err' as a vocal response out of your mouth trying to keep up with your brain. It's much more effective for you and your audience to allow the space, or pause. ^ Remember, everything you say and do is a choice, ^ so why would you choose to fill that space with the 'umm' or the 'err'? ^ Or filler words, for example: like, basically, you know, okay, look, right, and yeah.

When we have the courage to find the full stop, ^ we allow ourselves the space to think and **feel** and breathe the next thought before we deliver it. ^

It also gives the other person, or your audience, space to stay with you on your thought journey, ^ and to stay connected to you. ^ It's the difference between people feeling 'talked at' ^ and people feeling that you are truly talking with and to them in a dialogue. ^

Ultimately, it gives your audience space to understand and unpack what is important in what you are saying.

REFLECTIVE LEARNING EXERCISE

Ask someone you trust to do this exercise with you.

Tell them you are going to deliver a short anecdote or story. Keep it simple and under 2 minutes – for example, how you travel to work or you're favourite activity outside of work.

Ask them to raise a hand in front of you whenever they hear the end of a thought or a sentence from you, and then to put their hand down again after a second. When the hand goes up, you have to stop speaking, and wait for the hand to go back down before you start speaking your next thought. Use those moments when their hand is up to take the 'thinking breath'. Don't be waiting for their hand to go down again!

You may be surprised at how many times their hand goes up. You may find it distracting, as if someone is stopping you in your flow. But stay with the exercise. The other person will determine the pace of your delivery. It's as much about your audience's needs as it is your own.

Now swap over. Ask them to tell you a story for a couple of minutes. Do the same thing with your hand. You will quickly understand the need for space between the delivery and receiving of thoughts and how powerful it is for both parties. It creates connection, trust, and confidence.

Barack Obama is a master communicator. In his many speeches, you can see him leaving acres of space as he delivers his content. I never felt it meant he didn't know what he was talking about. As an audience we imbue the person who does have the courage to leave these spaces with high status, wisdom, and knowledge. This is the opposite of our feelings in the spotlight, giving the speech – our fear fills the space.

Give yourself the breath for the next thought. Do not hijack the conversation with an 'umm', as if you know what you are going to say next, when you don't.

The 'umm' is grabbing the conch shell without knowing what you are about to say.

Observe full stops when you speak, just as you would if it was punctuation on the page.

When I feel the anxiety bubbling away underneath, ^ I find a quiet private spot and I say this mantra out loud: ^

'This is my space. ^ I am not renting this space. ^ I'm not apologising for this space. ^ I own this space'. ^

GROUND

We talk about being grounded as a positive thing. Someone who is grounded – centred, stable, tethered, and focused – we observe as having presence.

The opposite is someone who is flighty, drifting, untethered, fidgety, or unfocused.

We trust someone more who appears grounded.

Even if they are not feeling grounded on the inside, as long as they show it I'm not going to see their fear. I'm not inside their head. I will only see someone who looks grounded.

Electricity needs to be earthed to be safe. It's the same with our nervous energy. It needs to be earthed or grounded. Then we can harness its power and direct it to support our presence. It creates trust for those around you when you are earthed.

When I am feeling anxious, I will physically centre myself.

Anxiety, fear, and stress are seeping into our machines or instruments all the time, like rust and dirt. Find those moments in the day when you can stabilise yourself again by connecting to the ground.

People sometimes say to me, 'But I like to walk and talk when I'm up on the podium. It helps me think. It feels more natural'.

My answer is this: moving is a great choice, as long as you find the earth again. If you are constantly moving, instead of finding stillness between movements, it can become distracting for an audience and for you, too.

It's the intention that drives any movement. If you want to inspire your audience, let the feeling of wanting to inspire direct your movement. Otherwise, you are just wandering.

A livewire can easily become very unfocused.

When you present to an audience, be the film of the book. You don't go to the movies to read the book!
JONATHAN GUY LEWIS

Performance, being animated, and taking your audience on a journey are key. Don't end up reading slides. You'll become a hostage to what you've written on them.

REFLECTIVE LEARNING EXERCISE

You can do this exercise either on your own or with a partner. It is particularly useful if you are coaching someone who is preparing to deliver an important speech or presentation.

Take two chairs, or stools, and place them between 6 and 8 feet apart in the space. Stand behind one of them. Feel the back of it or touch it. Hold it. Stand your ground. Resist the temptation to fidget or move from one foot to the other. Stay tall, with an engaged spine. Remember, every speech begins with an inbreath, otherwise nervous energy might well mean you start with an 'umm'! After you have delivered your opening thought, stop and walk to the other chair as you breathe and think of the next thing you want to say. You can only begin speaking that next thought when you have arrived behind this other chair and are standing your ground again. When you have finished delivering that second thought, find the full stop, breathe, and walk back to the first chair. When you are standing behind it again, you can begin speaking your third sentence, and so on until you have finished the speech.

Get into the habit of rehearsing in this way. It will soon become second nature. You will feel the coming together of space, ground, voice, body, and breath so that during the performance, you will have the choice to stand still or move, depending on the impact that you want to make.

People will forget what you say, forget what you did, but they never forget how you made them feel.
MAYA ANGELOU

INTENT

The recipe of intent.

Why do we say what we say? Why do we use those specific words?

What do we mean by intent?

Cover the list below before you carry on reading.

REFLECTIVE LEARNING EXERCISE

Write down as many words as you can that you associate with the word *intent*.

Then compare your list with mine.

Plan

Goal

Objective

Purpose

Outcome

Desire

Aim

Ambition

Aspiration

Direction

Course

Forethought

End

Consequence

The word missing from this list (and if you have it, congratulations, that's impressive) is…

Affect. Not effect, but affect.

An affect is something that you try to do to someone else or something else. A change, as in 'affect a change'.

To reassure someone.

To inspire the team.

To provoke a response.

To transform them through affecting an emotional response.

The reason why it's a *recipe of intent* is because, just like baking a cake, we need our main ingredients – butter, eggs, sugar, flour (gluten-free!) to create the sponge or base, otherwise it won't hold together.

But if we always bake sponge with nothing on top, no fillings or decoration, after a while we get bored of eating just sponge. We begin to crave something else with the cake.

It is the same with our intentions and communication style.

Often, we purely focus on updating or informing, authorising, or educating.

And these are our main ingredients, the rational, thinking intentions, but we struggle to make the content really land for people without the toppings and fillings: chocolate, fruit, cream, ginger, cinnamon. Feel free to add your personal favourites!

These are the emotional intentions which combine with feelings to create the compelling component. Our communication cake needs them.

And this is why, if asked what makes us human, emotions would be near the top of any list. Our emotions affect every aspect of our lives – every decision, big and small.

Darwin was fascinated by emotions. He concluded that they are there, in essence, to warn us very quickly whether a situation is safe or not. But often we have a complicated relationship with our emotions. We brand some as good and some as bad and others as somewhere in between.

The brain can be divided roughly into three areas: lizard brain, mammal brain, and human brain.

Lizard brain is the deepest structure. Its priority is to keep you alive. It involves itself with breathing, digestion, and keeping your heart beating. It doesn't really care what you think or feel.

Mammal brain is wrapped around the lizard brain. It's also known as the limbic system, and it is focused on your safety. This is the area of the brain that keeps track of your past pain and pleasure memories. All the mammal brain wants to do is to keep you safe at all times. So, if you have survived up to now by doing certain things, mammal brain will push you to keep repeating those same behaviours. Mammal brain hates any kind of change.

Human brain, or the neocortex (at the front of the brain), is the area that we can most easily and consciously access. It is the home of rational thought, learning, decision making, empathy, and creativity.

It's important to understand that these three areas of the brain don't always agree with each other. If the human brain wants to try out a new activity, the mammal brain might try and put the human brain in its place. It could induce anxiety and fear in order to persuade the human brain away from taking such a big risk.

The brain is also covered in neural networks that get stronger or weaker depending on how often they are used. The ones that get used repeatedly become strong 'neural highways'. These define our default thoughts and emotional responses – our personality. It's important to know that our neural pathways can be changed, even as we get much older. This is called neuroplasticity.

It is the prefrontal cortex that is involved with the regulating of emotions and decision-making. This is where we store our sense of self, our value system, and our self-control. We also use the prefrontal cortex to suppress emotions.

The amygdala is where we store our emotional memories. It assesses our environment for potential danger and produces the fear, anxiety, or anger that we might need to display in order to respond appropriately.

Our thalamus receives all the information from our senses – sight, touch, hearing, smell, and taste. And then it sends information to the different parts of the brain.

The hippocampus stores our memories. It stores the physical sensation of memories and emotions.

When we perceive something that makes us feel fear or anxiety, our thalamus sends a signal to the amygdala. The amygdala then checks with the hippocampus to see if we have previous memories that might tell us how to deal with it. If our hippocampus pings back painful emotional memories, we respond with fear and anxiety. Strong emotions can make our rational brain freeze or close down. The amygdala is much quicker than the rational brain to respond. The anxiety and fear leads to shallow breathing. This starves the brain of oxygen and leads to the areas of the brain not involved with survival taking a back seat. Rational thinking, empathy, and creativity all shut down.

Our thoughts can trigger emotional responses. If our human brain summons up a thought, or a memory, of a time when we felt shame or anger, for example, mammal brain can be triggered into producing a physical emotional reaction. We call these *feelings*.

Feelings are different from emotions, as they can be rationalised. An emotion happens very quickly; feelings are responses to our environment combined with our thoughts or inner beliefs about a situation. Feelings can therefore be managed more easily than emotions. We can question the feeling.

Emotional responses are rapid responses to specific things. Suppressing emotions when making decisions can have very negative consequences. It can lead to more indecision. If you don't take notice of your emotional response to things, it can lead you to a stressful state of 'analysis and paralysis', where you can't move forward. That is why it is never good when people say, 'Leave emotions out of this and stick to the facts'. We are not hardwired to do that.

If you try to deny the emotional aspect or dynamic in any conversation or meeting, or someone else does, it will always be the elephant in the room. It will leak out in some way. Presence means harnessing the facts and the feelings together – spinning two plates at the same time. It can be exhausting because it requires an energy of commitment and connection of being in the moment as much as possible with your communication.

But don't beat yourself up if you're not in the moment all the time. It's frankly impossible. Instead, think of it like surfing a wave.

When communication isn't congruent (matching), we notice it. We've all witnessed the person talking about how passionate they are, and yet they exude about as much energy and passion as a brick! It stops us focusing on what they are talking about – their content. It creates doubt and ambiguity. Or when we get distracted by someone's 'umm' or 'err', 'like' or 'you know' (the filler words) because they pepper their conversation with them like stepping-stones between their thoughts! It creates a fuzz, like looking at a Polaroid that's just out of focus. We end up counting the 'umms' rather than listening to the content.

A useful palette of emotional intentions to start with could include:

Excite
Inspire
Entertain
Flatter
Charm
Tempt
Cajole
Implore
Reassure

Placate

Challenge

Provoke

Scare

Shock

These are all useful intentions for your tool kit. Even scare and shock can be useful from time to time.

The key thing is to be aware of the two journeys you are creating with your content: the thought journey and the feelings and emotions journey in order to create and build trust.

For example, I need to inform you about something specific, but I will also try to inspire you as I inform you. And when you focus on an emotional intent with your content, you immediately become more congruent and specific with your communication.

You create more compelling narrative when you harness emotional as well as intellectual intentions.

REFLECTIVE LEARNING EXERCISE

Take a piece of content that you need to deliver or that you have recently delivered. Go through it and see if you can mark out the two journeys – the thinking and the feeling components. Where are you informing, updating, or educating? How could you add emotional intents underneath or alongside these? For example, is there an anecdote that can entertain as well as update? Is there a quote or statistic that can also inspire or excite?

Go further than you think you need to with emotional intents.

We tend to be conservative with the way we express them. Our herd or pack instinct tries to regulate what's acceptable to fit in, or rather not stand out. Often what's received by your audience is the watered-down, diluted version.

For example, we think we are being scintillating as we deliver the plan, but what is received by the audience is only mildly engaging.

Don't be afraid of turning your own dial up.

Sometimes during the courses I run at RADA Business, where everyone talks about work situations that have left emotional scars, that deeply buried hurt, anger, or fear can resurface. We then work through the conversation. We reenact it and rehearse how it could have had a better outcome for the participant. We look for the small body language leaks or emotions that are being sat on. We analyse the tone of voice and questioning tone that can seep in. With the skills that are learned earlier in the course, everyone is now equipped to become forensic in their analysis. It's very exciting. Everyone gets the chance to go through their own scene. Often the anger, hurt, pain, or fear that has been repressed seeps out in body language and the nonverbal subtext.

This exercise seems to really help unlock these deeply felt wounds. It helps the participant move on, as well as create catharsis and strength to do things differently next time.

And it is when we move on to rehearsing what I call the fantasy version of the meeting or the event that things get really interesting. We may have already gone over the scene a number of times, with the other participants offering redirection when necessary or sharing their own versions of that same scene. But this is the heightened version that the participant really wishes could have happened originally – what they really wanted to say but didn't. It's amazing what often comes out, how this releases the participant's shackles.

We create the conditions for our own success and failure in our heads.

JONATHAN GUY LEWIS

It's important, therefore, to replace the negative self-talk of 'I'm just not good at...', or 'I hate doing...', or 'I've never been good at...' or 'Please don't make me...' with 'I'm getting better at...', 'I'm really excited by...', or 'That's such an opportunity to...'

Positive self-talk works with the diaphragmatic breath to underpin the pillars of presence.

REFLECTIVE LEARNING EXERCISE

Take a piece of paper and write down a list of three things that you know you struggle with in terms of communication and presence – things that scare you or that make you run for the hills.

By each one of them, write a sentence that is positive, brave, and heartfelt. Then say that new sentence out loud three times. Make sure this sentence has your name in it, as something very powerful happens when we talk to ourselves positively using our own name.

Record it and play it back to yourself. Keep hold of the recording if you can. Every time you feel the self-doubt seep in, take out the recording and play it back to yourself.

For example:

'I hate speaking at the weekly team meetings. I'm not good at it. I hate everyone looking at me. I really wish I didn't have to do it. I'd avoid it if I could'.

Replace it with:

'(Your name), you're getting better at speaking at the weekly team meetings. It's an opportunity to share and connect, and I know they want me to succeed.

I really value hearing everyone else's stories'.

Optimising your communication style requires:

1. Eliminating *ambiguity* so that other people's perception of you matches your intent.

2. Creating *congruence* so that what you say is matched by how you say it.

If you say you're passionate about something, it needs to be reflected in what you're saying and how you express it. <u>You</u> have to 'turn the dial up' on connecting. And if your natural behavioural preference is more analytical or task-focused, you may find this harder to do because this isn't about the numbers or the plan.

REHEARSAL

It's important to get into the habit of doing something rather than nothing.

JONATHAN GUY LEWIS

We prepare our content to the nth degree; we tinker and rejig the slides in the deck we are about to present, sometimes literally minutes before delivering it. But how often do we make the time to run through it out loud?

If the answer is 'I don't have the time', then make the time to rehearse, not just prepare – even if it's only the first few minutes and the last few minutes of what you're going to talk about. What are you going to leave your audience thinking? How do you want them to feel as a result?

And as a personal favour to me, when you are rehearsing, don't refer to it as a 'dry run'. To me that implies a stale, dried-up, rigid version. Reframe it as a 'wet run'. All the pistons and cogs of your machine are going to have the oil they need to do the job.

Don't set yourself up for failure. Give yourself the best chance of success.

JONATHAN GUY LEWIS

If you've got a tricky conversation or one-to-one, make some time to practice the conversation with a colleague, friend, or peer. It might just save you time later. Better to find out in a rehearsal that your approach isn't landing than in the actual event!

You can save yourself time when you start rehearsing conversations, time that you may have spent correcting misunderstandings later.

'These new shoes pinch a bit. Should I buy them?'

It might not feel natural at first to try these techniques and pillars of presence. You may feel uncomfortable or self-conscious trying the exercises.

Replace the word *natural* with *habit*. We build habits over time, so when we start questioning the effectiveness of some of our habits, there might be resistance. Is it a security blanket? Maybe it's holding you back? Maybe the rational, processing brain is trying to protect its power. It doesn't want to give up control, but you might be missing an opportunity to expand your repertoire or add more tools in your tool kit.

Everything we do is a choice. Give yourself more choices.

JONATHAN GUY LEWIS

The work we do requires an element of jumping off into the unknown – to let go and release rather than control, which leads to overthinking. Too much emphasis or reliance on control, and the habit of control, can create a brittle rigidity and tightness. 'If I'm in control, I'll be okay'. But this control is often skin deep. It doesn't create stable foundations for you, and it doesn't allow for flexibility, ease, or flow in communication. The style can easily turn into 'My way or the highway'.

True presence does not come from knowing things, it comes from your gut, your centre, your flexibility, your ease, and your space because you've created a strong and stable foundation on which to communicate those things.

Give yourself permission.

ANONYMOUS

Permission to actively let go allows you to take the pressure off yourself. It can give you space to experiment, play, take a risk with your communication style, and surprise yourself.

If the 'bar of expectation' that you put on yourself is too high, it will eventually stop you from even trying. The perfectionist gene can stop you even having a go. So, you learn to fly under the radar. That way you don't risk making a mistake or getting it wrong. That's too scary and too painful to risk looking foolish. It eats away at confidence and therefore your presence.

CURIOSITY

Stay curious.

Often, we feel we add value when we go into solution mode. We then forget to stay curious.

Sometimes, you might then start solving the wrong problem. If you had dared to stay curious, you might have unearthed some buried treasure, which could mean answering an even bigger problem that someone didn't know about or was hidden from view.

Be more interested in others and want to know about their story and their journey more than your own.

Be a magpie. If something worked on you, take it and make it part of your tool kit – a story that moved you, from a leader who inspired you.

Be open to the possibility.

When you stay curious, people feel valued and affirmed. They will want to know more about you.

VISION

What is your purpose?

What is your 'why'?

This gives you the perspective to think broadly and strategically and helicopter above the day-to-day noise of communication, but also it gives you permission to focus on the detail when you need to.

It gives you a compass to find your way in the fog. You might not know the way exactly, but you may have a plan, goal, and vision. However, in the fog of not knowing and uncertainty, it can be daunting and scary to go on that journey. The fog can descend at any time, so having that compass can be a powerful aid to getting where you need to go.

It also means you have to be present in the now in order to read the compass.

A FINAL PIECE OF SCAFFOLDING AND A GIFT

The final thing I want to share with you in this chapter is the mantra or 'anchor' I use before I walk out onto a stage and into the spotlight. It works for me. I urge you to make your own, but I'll share my piece of scaffolding with you. And it's my gift to you if you want to borrow it.

I reach up with my hands high above my head and I lower an invisible bar (of expectation) to the floor, and I physically step over it, and I walk on to the stage. As I lower that bar and step over it, I say to myself out loud:

'I am good enough ^ and that is as good as it gets. ^ I have nothing to prove, which means there's nowhere to fall'. ^

It reminds me to be me.

Deep in my heart, and in good conscience, if I am true to myself and I have done the work, I know that that is enough to see me through. It creates stability for me. It reassures me. It reduces the negative noise, the clutter, and the demons in my head.

Will it be perfect?

Will I be perfect?

Will I get some of it wrong?

Probably.

But I know that I am good enough. And that is as good as it gets.

Summary

This chapter has explored:
- Pillars of presence. The scaffolding that you can employ to help you embrace your positive presence.
- Some of the challenges and barriers that get in the way – whether we put them there ourselves or we perceive others to have put them in our way.
- A number of exercises and tips to grow presence and authority.

Further Reading & Viewing

Amy Cuddy. Your body language may shape who you are (Amy Cuddy: Your body language may shape who you are | TED Talk) https://www.youtube.com/watch?v=Ks-_Mh1QhMc&t=2s.

Bolton R, Bolton DG. *People Styles at Work-and Beyond: Making Bad Relationships Good and Good Relationships Better.* Amacom Books; 2009.

Cameron J. *The artists way a course in discovering and recovering your creative self.* London: Pan; 1995.

Gladwell M. *Blink: the power of thinking without thinking.* Hachette Audio; 2010.

Mehrabian A, Ferris SR. Inference of attitudes from nonverbal communication in two channels. *Journal of consulting psychology.* 1967 Jun;31(3):248.

Sinek S. *Start with why: How great leaders inspire everyone to take action.* Penguin; 2009.

Van Der Kolk B. The body keeps the score. *Trauma.* 2003;2:50.

Wiseman R. *Rip It Up: Forget positive thinking, it's time for positive action.* Pan Macmillan; 2012.

CHAPTER 4

Creating Psychologically Safe Spaces: A Peer Coaching Approach

Pippa Gough

It is very well to say 'be prudent, be careful, try to know each other'. But how are you to know each other?

Florence Nightingale

CHAPTER OUTLINE

Clear, consistent, and compassionate leadership has never been more important to support nurses and other health staff in a time of extreme challenge. Knowing your own strengths and weaknesses as a leader and being able to flex your leadership style to respond appropriately is paramount. Coaching often challenges people in leadership positions to reflect on their approach. A useful question can be, "how might team talk about me when I am not around?" Responses may reveal clues about how a leader takes up their authority and what they role-model in their day-to-day work. Are they a listener, do they empower, are they comfortable with delegating, or are they someone who prefers to maintain power and gives instruction rather than consults? All of these behaviours are appropriate leadership responses but need to be applied with discretion in different situations at different times.

Regular one-on-one sessions with a coach is often seen as part of ongoing leadership development, but this may seem out of reach in times of crisis when conserving limited time and energy is privileged above life or career goals.

Peer coaching offers a different, more flexible approach which may create psychologically safe spaces for hard-pressed, emotionally challenged nurses and midwives and other health care staff and help contain the anxiety of the emotional, mental, and physical demands of caring work. This is done using a structured questioning/listening approach, allowing real-life work challenges to be explored and reframed so they may be tackled more effectively.

This chapter will explore what is meant by a psychologically safe space, a coaching approach, and the process of peer coaching. It will draw briefly on some of the theoretical underpinnings of the approach, including the importance of listening, giving attention, and allowing time to think (Kline, 1999). The chapter is based on learning by doing. Working with a partner and within a group of three, it will provide a number of practical exercises which allow you to experiment with the approach. To enhance the learning, it will encourage you to maintain reflective notes of your experience using Gibbs' reflective cycle (Gibbs, 1988).

- Clarify what is meant by psychologically safe spaces, a coaching approach, and peer coaching through applying these concepts in practice.
- Develop your 'learning by doing' through working in pairs and small groups with colleagues, using the structured questioning/listening approach, and writing reflective notes on the experience using Gibbs' reflective cycle.
- Identify key changes in leadership behaviour by maintaining reflective notes to track increased personal awareness using Gibbs' reflective cycle.
- Evaluate your personal effectiveness and personal power by recording examples of how you have experimented with this in your leadership practice and with what tangible impact.

What Is a Psychologically Safe Space?

Clarifying what this means to you:

This section will help you explore what feeling 'psychologically safe' at work means to you, through exercises aimed at:

- Developing your own ideas
- Drawing on your own experience
- Exploring some of the supporting literature

How very little can be done under the spirit of fear?

REFLECTIVE LEARNING EXERCISE

What does a psychologically safe space mean to you? Make a note of what occurs to you. Use words, pictures, or phrases. Examples of possible starter sentences are below:

When I'm in a psychologically safe space I feel . . .

The characteristics of a safe space are . . .

This space feels safe because . . .

My psychologically safe space is . . .

When I think of a safe space, I have a picture in my head which looks like this . . .

Many of your ideas emerging from the above exercise are reflected in the extensive supporting literature and research on the subject, which offers a range of explanations and defining attributes. For example:

- Turner and Harder (2018) explored the use of simulation as part of nurse education and found that learning was enhanced when students knew they could make a mistake without consequences.
- In focusing on psychological safety in health care teams, Edmondson et al. (2016) defined psychological safety as a belief that the context is safe for interpersonal risk taking, a belief that our voice is welcome and that we will not be judged, and a trust that our contribution will be welcomed, even if it turns out not to be right.

- Barbara Fredrickson, Kenan distinguished professor of psychology, University of North Carolina, Chapel Hill, known for her work on positivity, focuses on positive emotions such as trust, curiosity, confidence, and inspiration to broaden the mind and change behaviours in a lecture she gave in 2011 (https://www.youtube.com/watch?v=Z7dFDHzV36g. Accessed 27 June 2021). She suggests that we become more open-minded, resilient, motivated, and persistent when we feel psychologically safe.

This video of Amy Edmondson, Novartis professor of leadership and management at the Harvard Business School, talking about the importance of psychological safety at work is a useful summary of this concept (https://www.youtube.com/watch?v=eP6guvRt0U0. Accessed 26 May 2021).

Another important concept, drawing from psychodynamic theory, is the need for clarity around four things: boundaries, authority, role, and task (BART) (Green and Molenkamp, 2005) in order to contain anxiety and engender psychological safety.

- Boundaries can be seen as the safety container for group work by holding the 'task', the 'territory', and the 'time'.
- Authority involves the right to do the work, namely, the responsibility and the accountability for actions.
- Role concerns clarity about the roles people occupy. These can be achieved, acquired, assigned, or ascribed.
- Task can correspond to the mission of the organisation. It can also refer to the survival task of the group.

In summary, the defining attributes of a psychologically safe space include:

- Trust
- Confidentiality
- Respect
- Feeling confident
- Not feeling exposed or vulnerable
- No fear of criticism, retribution, or embarrassment
- Replacing conflict with support and challenge
- Being able to take risks, create, and experiment with new behaviours
- Development of a place where you can reflect and learn and be open to learning and view failure as a source of learning.

REFLECTIVE LEARNING EXERCISE

How might you go about creating a psychologically safe space with your team and/or colleagues? List five key things.

You will find it useful to read the publication by Michael West, Suzie Bailey, and Ethan Williams, published by the King's Fund in 2020, which you can find at this link: https://www.kingsfund.org.uk/sites/default/files/2020-09/The%20courage%20of%20compassion%20full%20report_0.pdf.

Your list may have included the following:

- Agreeing on a framework of ground rules
- Agreeing on confidentiality
- Clarifying roles and timing

- Listening without judging or criticizing
- Allowing time for reflection
- Allowing everyone to speak
- Encouraging everyone to speak
- Not interrupting people

WRITING REFLECTIVE NOTES

You will be asked to keep reflective notes as you work through the practical exercises set out in this chapter. Using the structure of Gibbs' Reflective Cycle (1988) is a helpful way to do this (Fig. 4.1). You may already be familiar with the process.

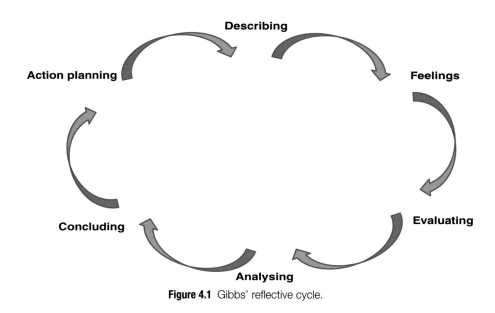

Figure 4.1 Gibbs' reflective cycle.

TABLE 4.1 ■ **The six steps of Gibbs' cycle**

Describing	What happened, what did you do, and what was the experience?
Feeling	What was the impact on you? How did you feel?
Evaluating	What went well, what could have been better, what was challenging for you, what was easy for you?
Analysing	What was actually happening? How do you understand what was going on?
Concluding	What did you learn about yourself and how you act in these situations?
Action planning	What might you do differently in the future as a result of this experience? What are your options now? What are your next steps?

The six steps of Gibbs' cycle are shown in Table 4.1.

Further reading on Gibbs' reflective cycle in nursing and professional development is given at the end of this chapter.

What Is a Coaching Approach?

Clarifying what this means to you:

- Developing your own ideas
- Drawing on your own experience
- Exploring some of the supporting literature
- Writing reflective notes

BRAINSTORMING EXERCISE

Whether you have coached others, have been coached, or neither, you likely have heard the word in a range of different applications, for example, sports coach, executive coach, life coach, retirement coach, and so on.

Write down what you know about 'coaching' and what you think a 'coaching approach' might mean.

What Is Coaching?

Coaching can be described as an approach that enables the client to determine their own goals and provokes learning that creates challenge and transformation. In this sense, coaching aims to be 'evolutionary'.

Rogers (2004) described six key principles that underpin coaching, namely:

- The client is resourceful.
- The coach's role is to release this resourcefulness.
- Coaching addresses the whole person – past, present, and future.
- The clients sets the agenda.
- The coach and the client are equal.
- Coaching is about change and action.

Executive coaching falls within this frame, defined by Management Futures (2016) as 'a powerful process designed to enhance leadership performance and effectiveness within an organisational context. We are clear that the primary purpose of coaching is to produce results. Coaching is an effective form of active learning, ideally dovetailing personal and organisational needs' (p 13).

A coaching approach describes a way of communicating well generally, particularly in relation to leading and managing, and it isn't restricted to a formal coach–client relationship.

KEY COACHING SKILLS FOR LEADERS

- Listening actively and giving 'generative attention' as described by Kline (1999).
- Asking powerful, exploratory, and open questions. The fundamental skill in using a coaching approach is asking questions because it provokes thought and assessment

from the other person. It allows them to develop different perspectives on a situation and reframe those issues they may be finding challenging so they might relate to them differently.

■ Clarifying goals and creating action plans that are practical and measurable.

Listening and Giving 'Generative Attention'

Kline (1999) developed the idea of a 'thinking environment' within which the quality of people's thinking is supported and enhanced by listening and not interrupting. Her work, based on allowing people 'time to think', explores the process and impact of allowing people to think uninterrupted whilst being held in the generative attention of others. This quality of attention, she argues, generates a quality of thinking which enables individuals to transform what they do and how they do it.

What Is a Powerful Question?

Powerful questions are ones that have a significant, positive impact on the quality and direction of a person's thinking about issues important to them. These questions are open (that is, they don't have a simple 'yes' or 'no' answer). They open up thinking rather than closing it down. Good exploratory questions usually start with a 'how' or a 'what', for example, 'How does that make you feel?' or 'How might you tackle this differently?' or 'What are your next steps?' Posing a question that starts with *why* can often make people feel defensive and may simply shut them down.

REFLECTIVE LEARNING EXERCISE

This is an exercise in listening and giving generative attention – one of the key skills in using a coaching approach. The exercise is drawn from the work of Nancy Kline and is known as 'thinking pairs'. It requires one person to think out loud whilst the other person listens without interrupting.

Work with a colleague. It's helpful to work through this exercise before moving on to the full peer-coaching exercise which is described in the next section.

You may find listening to someone who is thinking out loud, without interrupting them, somewhat challenging. You may also find the process of speaking your thoughts out loud whilst your colleague listens attentively (without interrupting you) equally testing. Give it a go and see how it feels.

Person A is going to be the 'listener' and Person B, the 'thinker'.

Person A will keep the time.

You are going to take 5 minutes each way.

■ Person A starts by saying the following to Person B (use the actual words):
  ■ 'I will not interrupt you'
  ■ 'I will ask you a question and will only ask you another question or respond to you if you invite me to do so'
  ■ 'What would you like to think about and what are your thoughts?'

■ Person B responds to the question and speaks (about anything they want) uninterrupted for 5 minutes.

- Person A listens, does not interrupt, and keeps their eyes on the thinker's eyes and their facial expression neutral. Try not to nod in approval, smile, or say anything at all.
- If Person B dries up, they ask for a second question.
- Person A asks the second question (use these actual words): 'What more do you think or feel or want to say?'
- If Person B dries up again then the second question is repeated.
- After 5 minutes, swap roles and repeat.

Once you have done this thinking pairs exercise, review the *process* with your partner. Tip: You will be tempted to get back into the *content* of what your thinking partner spoke about. If you find you have done this, move back into discussion of *process:*

- How did you create a psychologically safe space at the outset of the process?
- What did having time to think out loud, without interruption feel like?
- What was it like listening without interrupting or adding in your comments?
- What was challenging?
- What surprised you?
- What did you enjoy?

On your own, reflect further on the process and write down your views and insights about this approach using Gibbs' Reflective Cycle (Gibbs 1988).

A Peer-Coaching Approach

Putting into practice your learning about:
- Creating a psychologically safe space
- Experiencing being a 'client' and a 'peer coach' as part of a peer-coaching approach
- Reflecting on your experience

You have already thought about what it means to create a psychologically safe space. It is essential that for peer-coaching to be helpful, it must feel safe for all participants. Before undertaking the peer-coaching exercise set out below, it will be important to discuss with your colleagues what will help each other feel psychologically safe and agreeing a framework of ground rules. By so doing, you can cocreate with your colleagues not only a boundaried, confidential space where you can reflect on your leadership style and challenges but also a place of emotional refuge and sanctuary.

AIMS OF PEER COACHING

- Using a structured questioning/listening approach that allows real-life work challenges to be explored and reframed, in a safe space, so they may be tackled more effectively
- Helping a colleague learn more about a work issue that they find problematic so that they can think about how they might behave differently
- Developing coaching/consultancy skills. That is, the establishment, management, and conclusion of a relationship designed to help another explore what is problematic without telling them what to do
- Increasing understanding of how one learns

You will find it helpful to watch with your colleagues this video of a Zoom peer-coaching session before engaging in your own round of peer coaching. https://www.youtube.com/watch?v=H-AsZCnK5Bo.

BRIEFING FOR THE PEER-COACHING LEARNING EXERCISE

The approach we are proposing is based on asking questions. Questions that encourage a deeper exploration of what is going on, which can lead to alternative ways of behaving.

Work in groups of three. When you meet for the first time, agree on any ground rules and the running order. Each person in the group has the opportunity to take up the role of client and peer coach.

Client: The client presents a real and current work problem or situation that is not neatly defined.

Two peer coaches: The peer coach's role is to establish a supportive and challenging coaching relationship to help the client develop an understanding of what is going on and think about how to improve things. One of you is responsible for time keeping and managing the process and the structure of the session.

To help you frame powerful, open questions, a list of useful questions is included at the end of this section.

The Structure (35 Minutes)

Time (Minutes)	Activity
4	The client sets out the problem without interruptions.
2	When they have finished, one of the peer coaches summarises what they have heard without evaluation.
	The peer coach can also describe (briefly) their initial emotional/feeling response to the client's situation, without entering into conversation or passing judgement (e.g. 'Listening to you made me feel tired/happy/frustrated/angry/tearful/relieved/overwhelmed'.)
5	The peer coaches ask *clarifying questions* to ensure their own understanding of the situation (e.g. 'How many in your team?' or 'How long have you worked there?'
10	The peer-coaches ask *open questions* that deepen the client's description of what is going on. A collection of useful and powerful open questions for you to experiment with are given under Further Reading at the end of this chapter.
5	The peer coaches develop their explanations of what is going on and ideas about behaving differently.
	The client listens, trying to notice how they are responding in terms of their thoughts and feelings. (The client might want to write these down.)
4	The client summarises how they are thinking and feeling about their issue, without interruption, and if possible says something about how they might now behave.
5	Review of the process. The group reflects on how they managed *the process* of the session. Don't get back into the *content*.

REFLECTIVE LEARNING EXERCISE

Using Gibbs' reflective cycle, think through your experience. Consider:

- What questions this process raises for you?
- What do you remain curious about?
- What was challenging?
- What did you find comfortable/easy?

- What was it that helped you feel comfortable/made it easy?
- How might you apply these skills at work?

Examples of Useful Questions

- What result do you want?
- What is your biggest difficulty or problem?
- How do you feel about this situation?
- What would you do differently?
- What do you want the other person to do differently?
- What judgements are you making about the other person and/or the situation?
- How do you know this?
- Can you explain that further?
- What would make the situation better?
- How does the situation affect you?
- What don't you know about the situation?
- What is the most extreme measure you could take?
- What is the best possible outcome from this situation?
- What's the issue?
- What makes it an issue now?
- How important is it on a 1 to 10 scale?
- Who owns the issue/problem?
- What have you already tried?
- What's the ideal outcome?
- What is standing in the way of the ideal outcome?
- What's going right here (even if it is only a little bit)?
- What are the options for action here?
- What criteria would you use to judge the options?
- Which option seems the best one against those criteria?
- So what's the first/next step?
- When will you take it?

What Are My Next Steps?

Your skills at asking and refining powerful, open questions will increase exponentially with every session of peer coaching you participate in. You will find as well that whether you are the client or the peer coach your learning will be the same. As you help the client explore aspects of their behaviour, so you will be asking similar questions of yourself and deepening the understanding of how you are relating to some of the challenges you face.

Try and use the peer-coaching approach regularly with your colleagues. It can provide a vital pressure release for you all as well as powerful learning about your leadership and how this can be done differently and more effectively.

Summary

Peer coaching offers a different, more flexible approach, which may serve to create psychologically safe spaces for hard-pressed, emotionally challenged nurses and midwives and other health care staff. It can help contain the anxiety of the emotional, mental, and physical demands of caring work. The process uses a structured questioning/listening approach, allowing real-life work challenges to be explored and reframed so they may be tackled more effectively.

The objectives of this chapter were to:

- Clarify what is meant by psychologically safe spaces, a coaching approach, and peer coaching and applying these concepts in practice.
- Develop your 'learning by doing' through working in pairs and small groups with colleagues, using the structured questioning/listening approach and writing reflective notes on the experience using Gibbs' reflective cycle.
- Identify key changes in leadership behaviour by maintaining reflective notes to track increased personal awareness using Gibbs' reflective cycle.
- Evaluate your personal effectiveness and personal power by recording examples of how you have experimented with this in your leadership practice and its tangible impact.

The chapter has explored what is meant by a psychologically safe space, a coaching approach, and the process of peer coaching. It has drawn on some of the theoretical underpinnings of the approach, including the importance of listening, giving attention, and allowing time to think.

The chapter is based on learning by doing. Working with a partner and within a group of three, it provided a number of practical exercises which has enabled you to experiment with the approach. To enhance the learning, you were encouraged to maintain reflective notes of your experience and learning using Gibbs' reflective cycle (Gibbs, 1988).

References

Edmondson, A.C., Higgins, M., Singer, S., Weiner, J., 2016. Understanding psychological safety in health care and education organizations: A comparative Perspective. Res. Human Dev. 13 (1), 65–83. doi: 10.1080/15427609.2016.1141280. https://www.tandfonline.com/doi/full/10.1080/15427609.2016.1141280. Accessed 30 May 2021.

Edmondson, A., 1999. Psychological safety and learning behavior in work teams. Adm. Sci. Q. 44 (2), 350-383. Sage Publications, Inc. on behalf of the Johnson Graduate School of Management, Cornell University. Stable URL: http://www.jstor.org/stable/2666999. Accessed 4 October 2016; https://content.tcmediasaffaires.com/LAF/lacom/psychological_safety.pdf. Accessed 3 April 2021.

Gibbs, G., 1988. *Learning by Doing: A Guide to Teaching and Learning Methods*. Oxford Further Education Unit, Oxford.

Green, Z.G., Molenkamp, R.J., 2005. The BART system of group and organizational analysis: Boundary, authority, role and task. https://www.researchgate.net/publication/277890284_Boundary_Authority_Role_and_Task. Accessed 30 May 2021.

Kline, N., 1999. *Time to Think*. Hachette Book Group, New York.

Management Futures, 2016. Intensive coaching skills programme. MF, London.

Rogers, J., 2004. *Coaching Skills. A Handbook*. Open University Press, Milton Keynes.

Turner, S., Harder, N., 2018. Psychological safe environment: A concept analysis in simulation. Nursing 18, 47–55. https://www.nursingsimulation.org/action/showPdf?pii=S1876-1399%2817%2930146-9. Accessed 26 May 2021.

Further Reading (On Reflective Cycles)

Barksby, J., et al., 2015. A new model of reflection for clinical practice. *Nursing Times* 111 (34/35), 21–23.   https://www.nursingtimes.net/roles/nurse-educators/a-new-model-of-reflection-for-clinical-practice-17-08-2015/. Accessed 27th June 2021.

Bolton, G., Delderfield, R., 2018. *Reflective Practice: Writing and Professional Development*, fifth ed. Sage, Los Angeles, London, New Dehli, Singapore.

Schon, D., 1984. *The Reflective Practitioner: How Professionals Think in Action*. Basic Books Inc, USA.

University of Edinburgh, 2020. Gibbs reflective cycle as part of the online Reflection Tool Kit. https://www.ed.ac.uk/reflection/reflectors-toolkit/reflecting-on-experience/gibbs-reflective-cycle. Accessed 27 June 2021.

CHAPTER 5

Leading in Anxious Times

Amy Hart

CHAPTER OUTLINE

This chapter aims to break down the job of leadership to make sense of the challenges of leading in these anxious times.

In this chapter we recognise how context can drive anxiety and how that can drive behaviours in ourselves and others.

It offer some contemporary thinking about leadership while the world adapts around us.

It offer some tips and thoughts for individuals, teams, and organisations to consider.

OBJECTIVES

- To consider the job of leadership.
- To consider the challenges of leading in anxious times.
- To consider the challenges of leading in anxious times.
- To understand the impact of effective leadership in organisations.

Introduction

It is a privilege to write a chapter for the Florence Nightingale Foundation because it is a moment to reflect, when the world is full of challenges, on the importance of the role of nursing.

Before we start defining the job of leadership, in the next chapter, it seems prudent to recognise the phenomenal leadership provided by Florence Nightingale, as current today as it was in the 1850s, best summarised by her quote: *'To be "in charge" is certainly not only to carry out the proper measures yourself but to see that everyone else does so too'*. We interpret this to mean that Florence identified the importance of how you model leadership to people. What people will notice about leaders is that leadership is both a gift and a responsibility.

The Job of Leadership

There is much written about leadership skills, leadership approaches, and leadership behaviour. However, the job/framework of leadership is rarely defined in a way that enables it to be clear and understandable. The Centre for Creative Leadership (CCL) defines leadership as a 'social process that enables individuals to work together to achieve results'. The CCL describes the Direction, Alignment and Commitment (DAC) framework of leadership, meaning that whether you are within a team, workgroup, division, or entire organisation, leadership must include three elements: direction, alignment, and commitment. The CCL describes *direction* as agreement on what the collective are trying to achieve, *alignment* as effective coordination and integration of the different aspects of the work so they fit together in service of the shared direction, and *commitment* as people who are making the success (not just individual success) a personal priority.

According to the CCL, the absence of these three elements within organisations results in an impact on organisational effectiveness. They cite examples where people are unclear about how their work fits with the organisational goals, or how people jump into tasks and projects without connecting it to the work of others. The result is the unnecessary duplication of effort and suboptimal outcomes. Ensuring DAC will enable individuals and teams to work in true service of the organisational requirements and ambition. This is more deeply enhanced when individuals believe the organisational mission aligns with their personal mission.

The chart below shows the impact/cause of having or not having DAC in place for organisations:

If you are a leader looking at this table, ask yourself three key questions:

1. Do I always set direction for my people?

2. Do I align my activities and encourage others to do so?

3. How do I know my people are as committed and engaged in the work as needed?

If the answer is yes to any of the questions above, ask yourself, 'How could I do this better?' If the answer is no, ask yourself, 'What's stopping me?'

The second consideration for leaders, when thinking about their leadership job, is to consider the early work from the global HR consultancy, Hay Group (now Korn Ferry), on organisational climate, described as 'how it feels to work in a particular environment'. This research showed that organisational climate can directly impact people's performance by 30%. The climate work built on the early work of David McClellan, 1961, who proved that human beings operate with three motives: (1) achievement, based on personal performance; (2) affiliation, the desire for close, warm relationships; and (3) power, based on the desire to influence and work through others. The effect of this on organisational climate, then and now, is that people need to feel they are achieving, valued, and connected to others – interdependent in their accomplishment. The expression 'interdependent in their accomplishment' is a sentiment expressed by Professor Michael West when he looked at effective health care teams in his 2000 research.

The work of David McClellan could be a tool to help you consider your team's commitments and engagement in their work. Dolan and Lingham have created a web-based self-assessment that identifies the three motives for people (https://app.myeducator. com/reader/web/885/chapter3/h84ju/).

Our work with National Health Service (NHS) individuals, teams, and organisations has provided insights into what affects energy and motivation. Interestingly, we have observed a stage of development for senior leaders where their motivation is challenged as they need to reimagine what performance means and shift from personal performance to performing through people. In Good to Great, former Stanford business professor Jim Collins offers a primer on turning the average into the exceptional. Through detailed case studies of companies that were seen as three times more successful, Collins presents the key factors that separate merely good organisations from great ones, specifically relating to the point about reimagining performance. Collins' work highlights what he calls 'level 5 leadership'. Level 5 leaders display a powerful mixture of personal humility and indomitable will. They're incredibly ambitious, but their ambition is first and foremost for the cause, for the organisation and its purpose, not themselves.

Collins' work is significant to our work; we know that senior leaders who are seen as credible and trusted are those who base their decisions on the 'right thing to do given the circumstances, without losing sight of the future impact'. What this means in practice is that these leaders rarely think about how a decision may reflect on them personally, rather they are driven by making the right decision regardless of the personal consequences.

Leading When Feeling Anxious

So, having explored what the job of leadership is, this next section is best captured by the quote from Antarctic explorer Ernest Shackleton, who experienced untold adversity on the Antarctic expedition of 1914. He said that 'if you're a leader, a fellow that other fellows look to, you've got to keep going'. This can be incredibly daunting if you are the one that people are looking towards. There is an understanding that Shackleton enabled his followers to believe that he had a map and a plan when, in fact, he was making it up as he led others across the Antarctic, trusting his instinct, listening to all his senses to guide his team forward. There are similarities to the challenges of the global COVID-19 pandemic in 2020 and 2021.

From the conversations we have had with over 500 United Kingdom (UK) health care professionals, we understand that many have led whilst managing their own anxiety. We don't know for sure when pressure and uncertainty becomes anxiety, but we do know that anxiety is a normal emotion to experience. Physiologically, anxiety can mean that individuals experience a rush in adrenalin that leaves them instinctively responding with the primitive survival response of fight or flight or freeze.

Understanding the impact of anxiety on performance dates back to the work of Yerkes and Dobson, who discovered that too much or too little arousal can have an effect on different types of athletic performance tasks. While a basketball player or baseball player might need to control excessive arousal to concentrate on successfully performing complex throws or pitches, a track sprinter might rely on high arousal levels to motivate peak performance. In such cases, the type of task and complexity of the task plays a role in determining the optimal levels of arousal. This is interesting when considering the complexity of the tasks required of a leader in health care.

The 2020 Harvard Business Review (HBR) article *Leading Through Anxiety* focuses mostly on the effect of the global COVID-19 pandemic impact on leaders. It concludes that when anxiety is channelled effectively, it can have a positive impact on performance: 'In an economic crisis, the anxiety that keeps us up at night may help us fathom a solution to keeping our businesses open. But left unchecked, anxiety distracts us, zaps our energy, and drives us to make poor decisions. Anxiety is a powerful enemy, so we must make it our partner'. We understand this to mean that feeling anxious can either overwhelm or focus us. In the HBR article, Alice Boyes elaborates on leaders who fail to realise they are anxious, therefore leaving the anxiety 'unchecked'. Such leaders may respond to anxiety by trying to be more perfect and more in control, according to Boyes. In many societies those behaviours are rewarded and thought of as a good work ethic, but often perfectionism and overwork only cause further anxiety in ourselves and others. This reflection reminds us of the importance of self-awareness and self-diagnosis when we are anxious and the ability to consider what this could mean for the impact of our behaviour on ourselves and others.

Use this checklist, compiled from a variety of sources, to help ask several reflective questions about anxiety. These questions are especially helpful when we are starting to feel anxious:

- Why am I feeling anxious?
- What evidence do I have that this is going to be an issue?
- What is the best, worst, and most likely scenario to play out?
- Based on the past, how am I likely to end up coping with this?
- What is in my control that I can do something about?
- Who can help me work this through?

Effective Leadership

Effective leadership is a concept covered by many leadership theorists, academics, and people in business. Most people who enter a leadership position hope to be effective and may fear being seen as ineffective. This can be especially true when attempting to lead under pressure and uncertainty. In this section, we offer a reminder of what effective leadership is and what impact it can make on organisations.

A good place to start thinking about effective leadership is the learnings and reflections of Sir Robert Francis, whose review followed the Mid Staffordshire Trust scandal where between 400 and 1200 patients died as a result of poor care over the 50 months between January 2005 and March 2009. The Francis report was published based on a public inquiry into poor care at the Mid Staffordshire NHS Foundation Trust. The inquiry focused on failings within the Trust itself and concluded that patients were routinely neglected by an organisation which had lost sight of its fundamental responsibility to provide safe care. Of the 290 recommendations contained within the report, a significant section is related to leadership.

The Francis report identified the need for significant culture change within the NHS and was clear in stating that leadership creates culture. Francis placed an emphasis on strong leadership at every level of the NHS, and he called for openness, transparency, and candour. It was an important reminder of what can happen when, to quote John F Kennedy, 'The only thing necessary for the triumph of evil is for good men to do nothing'.

What we understand from this quote and its application to the NHS is that leaders in the NHS need to set and live by the culture and expectations that deliver the best care because when this fails it impacts many lives. This reminds us of the importance of the leadership role in healthcare. In 2014 Professor Michael West et al. wrote a paper describing the response to the Francis review entitled 'Developing Collective Leadership for Healthcare'. This article creates a context for leaders to lead in a way that ensures caring cultures are created, nurtured, and maintained. In the article, collective leadership is defined as 'everyone taking responsibility for the success of the organisation as a whole – not just for their own jobs or work area'.

The article describes how collective leadership relates to a culture of caring by suggesting that senior leaders must understand the leadership practices and behaviours needed to nurture a caring culture (pg 8) (West et al 2014). Understanding culture alone is insufficient. Conscious, deliberate attention must be paid to enabling people at every level within the organisation to adopt leadership practices that nurture the cultures the NHS requires.

For collective, distributed leadership (and followership), all staff must be engaged. It further adds that 'if we want staff to treat patients with respect, care and compassion, all leaders and staff must treat their colleagues with respect, care and compassion'. From this, we identify two important ways a leader can create a caring culture. First, through genuine staff engagement, and second, how leaders role-model caring, respectful, and compassionate behaviour to the people they lead.

West developed a checklist when thinking about compassionate leadership, demonstrating compassion when dealing with a patient and family and when working within the organisation.

So, how might you as a leader ensure that you engage with your staff and role-model the right behaviours? We believe this is especially difficult when leaders are under pressure and or are anxious. Our final section offers some tips on how leaders can still deliver the best outcomes even when anxious or uncertain.

Tips and Thoughts

This final section is based on our knowledge and understanding of current leadership theory and best practice and our experience of the reality of leading in the NHS. We know and understand that services are very often stretched, under-resourced, politically driven, and challenged. We also know that leadership creates a culture, and culture is more important and impactful than any written strategy. Culture drives performance which can be positive or negative. What we offer below is taken from a variety of sources already used and our own experience of working in and with the NHS.

Understand the Context in Which You Operate

Leaders who understand their context are more likely to be better aligned to the service/mission of their organisation and its key stakeholders. Knowing the direction and priorities of an organisation or system makes it easier to provide day-to-day leadership in service of organisational strategy, understanding your context is linked to the next tip of understanding the job of leadership. The practical application of understanding your context could be do all or some of the following:

- Attend any annual general meetings your organisation holds; you can learn a lot about how the organisation is working to serve your community.
- Even if you have been in the organisation for several years, act like an inductee, read board papers, strategic documents, and any information that helps you understand the organisational mission.
- Be curious and open to understanding as much as possible about what is important regarding the environment you work in.

Understand the Job of Leadership

The job of leadership at any level is to create direction, align the activities, and inspire your staff. This can be further enhanced if, like West teaches us, we operate in an environment with compassion and true genuine staff engagement. The practical application of understanding the job of leadership could be to do all or some of the following:

- No matter what day-to-day, week-to-week, or month-to-month activity you are doing, begin with the end in mind and act accordingly.
- Educate, enthuse, and, if necessary, enforce the direction of travel to keep you and your staff on track.
- Help your team align their activities towards the direction and maximise your coaching skills by asking your staff questions to help them consider how their work fits.

Know Yourself

We all respond to stress and pressure in differing ways. Understanding our individual personality traits, preferences, and leadership styles enables us to make decisions about the leadership choices we make. Leaders need to know when they are operating outside their comfort zone, what this means for their own personal resilience, and how to put the right support in place. Teams who reflect on their performance perform better than teams who don't. The practical application of knowing yourself could be do all or some of the following:

- Invest in personal development to help understand yourself as much as possible. There are many psychometrics and personality questionnaires that can provide a helpful insight into our preferences and ways of working.
- Role-model the culture you want to create, and think about your own preferences and when you need to work out of preference to create the right culture.
- Give and receive feedback: What is it like working for you? How do you know if you are doing a good enough job?

Know Your People

Your people include more than those who report directly to you – this statement applies in a 360-degree way. Knowing your direct team members is really important; however, it is also important to understand your manager(s) and colleague(s), as influencing others is a key leadership skill. Here are some practical applications of knowing your people:

- Prioritise genuine staff engagement – the answers sit with the people you lead. You don't have to have all the answers. Ask people what they know, think, and feel and what to do to improve things and act on it.
- Manage your manager – helping your manager achieve is key to your success. Work with your manager to find shared objectives and ways of working.
- Build relationships across the organisation – be open to learning from others and encourage cross-organisational work to help minimise tribalism and encourage organisational change.

Create and Maintain Balance

In short, work-life balance is the state of equilibrium where a person equally prioritises the demands of one's career and the demands of one's personal life. As with any role that we inhabit, it is important to find balance between our primary and secondary roles, and our leadership role is no different. The practical application of maintaining balance could be do all or some of the following:

- People will follow what you say and what you do. If you are asking your staff to take time off, you need to do so, too.
- Prioritise the balance that you need to enable you to be at your best when you are in your leadership role – this will depend on your personality and other factors.
- Set boundaries for yourself and stick to them.

Concluding this chapter, we quote Florence again: 'Live life when you have it, life is a splendid gift – there is nothing small about it'. We would apply this to leadership: 'Leadership is a splendid gift – there is nothing small about it!'

References

Aaron-Mele, M. 2020 Leading Through Anxiety. Harvard Business Review. Available: https://hbr.org/2020/05/leading-through-anxiety?msclkid=7fcf28a6b0bf11ec9491445 2c4ec40c6 Accessed 31/03/2022

Centre for Creative Leadership, (2020) Direction + Alignment + Commitment (DAC) = Leadership. Available: https://www.ccl.org/articles/leading-effectively-articles/make-leadership-happen-with-dac-framework/ Access: 31/03/2022.

Collins J., 2001. *Good to great, first ed*. Random House.

Freedom to Speak Up (2015) An independent review into creating an open and honest reporting culture in the NHS. http://freedomtospeakup.org.uk/the-report/.

Vielmetter, G. (2008) How leaders create engaged performanceand how to measure it. http://drber.com/d/2e447fc78e55460a9ca3ffc8ff3cb01a/files/Georg%20Vielmetter.pdf.

West et al (20014) Developing Collectives Leadership for Healthcare. The Kings Fund. http://www.ctrtraining.co.uk/documents/DevelopingCollectiveLeadership-KingsFundMay2014.pdf.

Yerkes R.M., Dodson J.D., 1908. The relation of strength of stimulus to rapidity of habit-formation. *Journal of Comparative Neurology and Psychology* 18 (5), 459–482. Reprinted by Green C.D. Classics in the History of Psychology. An Internet Resource. York University, Toronto, Ontario.

Further Reading/Resources (on Leadership and Effectiveness)

Arbinger Institute, 2016. *The anatomy of peace*. Penguin.

Brown B., 2018. *Daring Greatly*. Penguin.

Covey S., 2004. *7 habits of highly effective people*. Simon & Schuster Ltd.

Daniel Pink (motivation) https://www.youtube.com/watch?v=TopBJ7fAIgE.

Affina Organisation Development Ltd. (Team Working). www.affinaod.com.

Michael West: Compassionate and inclusive leadership. https://www.youtube.com/watch?v=RrPm Mwg9X8s.

RSA ANIMATE: Drive: The surprising truth about what motivates us. https://www.youtube. com/watch?v=u6XAPnuFjJc&t=3s.

Simon Sinek - Do you love your wife? https://www.youtube.com/watch?v=TopBJ7fAIgE.

Simon Sinek (leadership) https://www.youtube.com/watch?v=XGQo-Vge-WU.

CHAPTER 6

Gaining Political Acumen, Having Influence, and Making Change Happen

Catherine Eden

Were there none who were discontented with what they have, the world would never reach anything better.

Florence Nightingale

CHAPTER OUTLINE

Since the time of Florence Nightingale, nurses and midwives have been involved in campaigning for change, for their professions, for wider society, for organisations, and for the patients that they support. For many, words such as politics, campaigning, and influencing are daunting ones. However, armed with a few tips, tools, and a look at some successful examples of nurses thinking politically and influencing effectively, there are things that every nurse and midwife can do with more confidence and with a greater chance of success.

This chapter will explore the history of campaigning and political involvement by nurses and midwives since the time of Florence Nightingale and hear the perspectives of nurses who have become politicians. It will give some very practical tips and ideas for increasing political acumen and putting ideas into practice. It is a chapter very much grounded in practical experience, rather than academic theory, and it will leave the reader with increased political understanding and tools to influence more successfully and with more confidence to believe that change is possible.

OBJECTIVES

- Understand how the history of nurses campaigning for change and influencing policy and practice impacts today's nurses and midwives.
- Reflect on your own political astuteness and how you can improve it.
- Build on successful campaigns and approaches in the past: what works, what doesn't work.

- Apply approaches for planning change, giving you the best chance of success.
- Consider specific approaches for successfully working with elected politicians, local and national.
- Develop confidence to make change happen.

A Brief History of Influencing for Change by Nurses: Discontented Nurses Have Changed the World

Florence Nightingale and her campaigning for change is well documented, but some of her achievements have also set the standard for those who have followed her into the nursing profession and who want to campaign for change.

Having returned to England from the Crimean War and becoming acutely aware of the role poor sanitation and conditions had on the soldiers, Florence campaigned for a Royal Commission into the state of the army in India. She gathered facts and analysed the data, publishing her book *Observations on the Sanitary State of the Army in India* in 1863, in which she made the case that 'sanitary reform must be generally introduced into India for the civil, as well as the military portion of the population'.

Prior to 1865, 'nurse in workhouses were mainly unqualified and illiterate women, meaning that reading medicine bottles, among other things, was impossible. Together with William Rathbone, an English philanthropist, Florence sent 12 qualified nurses and 18 probationers from the Nightingale Training School for Nurses to the Liverpool Workhouse in 1865. This led to workhouse nursing reforms across the United Kingdom.

The Metropolitan Poor Bill of 1867 marked the first acknowledgement in English law that the state had a responsibility to provide hospitals for the poor and an important first step towards the emergence of the National Health Service 80 years later. In addition to workhouse infirmaries, the Bill also provided for the establishment of asylums for the sick and poor. Florence campaigned for improvements to the Metropolitan Poor Bill, including a centralised administration system and for workhouse nurses to be paid 'the market price for their labour'.

Having seen the lack of support and health services for pregnant women and those giving birth in India, Florence wrote to the Duke of Westminster in 1896 describing her plan to 'introduce in India native women health missioners to bring health among native rural mothers, by showing them what to do as friends'. Florence had recognised the importance of women being given support by those who shared their religion, customs, and culture, rather than support imposed by outsiders.

But as modern-day nurses wanting to change the world for the better (maybe starting locally), there are many other inspirational nurse leaders on whose shoulders you can stand and from who to be inspired:

Mary Seacole, who honed her nursing skills in the Caribbean where she was born, then close to the fighting in the Crimean war, exhibited the skills that continue to be needed by nurses who are wanting change for their patients, communities, and profession; good citizenship and achievement (she remains one of history's greatest figures) hold true today.

In mid-1800s America, Dorothea Dix played an instrumental role in the founding and expansion of more than 30 hospitals for the treatment of people who were mentally ill. She was a leading figure in national and international movements that challenged the idea that people with mental ill-health could not be cured or helped.

Lillian Wald, the founder of public health nursing, worked in New York in the late 19th and early 20th centuries. She believed that every resident was entitled to equal and fair health care regardless of their social status, socioeconomic status, race, gender, or age. She argued that everyone should have access to at-home-care and that all should have access to care, no matter their ability to pay, through the Henry Street Settlement that she founded and worked from. She used the term *public health nurse* to describe nurses whose work is integrated into the community.

In the 1930s, Australian nurse Elizabeth Kenny disagreed that polio patients should have their limbs cast, instead using warm compresses and a range of gentle motion that she noticed much improved results. Her work led to the founding of physiotherapy as a discipline.

In the 1950s in Essex, Sister Jean Ward discovered that babies with jaundice could be cured after being put outside in the sun for a few hours, beginning the use of photo-therapy for neonatal jaundice.

Dame Cicely Saunders founded the hospice movement and palliative care as a discipline, opening the first hospice in London in 1967.

In more modern times, many of the nursing profession's achievements have focussed on the development of the profession, whilst at the same time supporting campaigns for social change. In the last 50 years, nursing has become a degree-holding profession, nurses have increased their powers to prescribe drugs, and the professional roles of nurses have developed to give us advanced nurse practitioners, consultant nurses, and nurse associates. The profession has also campaigned for improved pay and conditions for nurses and an improved National Health Service (NHS) in addition to in which nurses and midwives want to work.

Gaining Political Acumen

Put simply, politics in all its forms is about, getting things done ', but it holds a lot of fear for many people. However, with some thought about the approach you take, combined with good preparation using the ideas that follow, you will stand a much better chance of being successful in whatever you want to change or get done.

First, some political acumen is helpful. It's not something that you can acquire through reading along, but it comes through observing and putting into practice behaviours and approaches towards a situation. It can be learned through observation of others, analysing why an approach to a particular situation was successful or not, and using some tested techniques to help. Cultivating your political antennae is vital for nurses and midwives who want to develop their political leadership skills both inside and beyond their organisations.

In 1987, Simon Baddley and Kim James wrote an academic paper *Owl, Fox, Donkey or Sheep: Political Skills for Managers*, which describes a model to assess and develop political astuteness. It focusses on two dimensions: the skill of 'reading' the politics of an organisation and the skills an individual brings. They characterise these approaches into four types of behaviour: innocent, inept, clever, and wise, which an individual may adopt in different situations and to which each of the animals in the paper's title were assigned (Baddley & James, 1987).

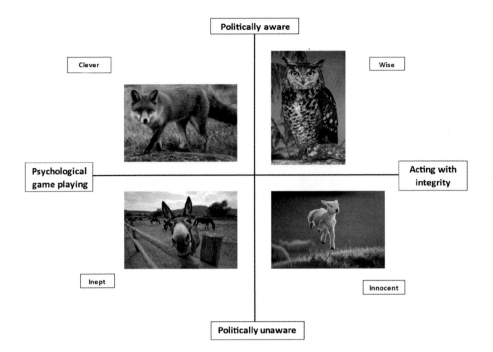

Looking at the diagram where do you think you are in the quadrant? Where are the people with whom you have interacted, maybe even tried to influence? For nurse and midwifery leaders who want to be successful influencers, being a bit 'more owl' is probably what you are aiming for.

It is also worth thinking about your spheres of influence, which may be more numerous than you think. There are so many places where nurses and midwives can have an impact, but in order to do that, you will need to understand the politics and potential of each sphere.

Organisation: the place(s) where you work

Local: your organisation plus other local interested parties, including local government, voluntary and community sector, and patient groups

System: local plus (usually) wider geography and health and care 'system'

Profession: professional bodies, colleges, regulators, and trades unions

National: wider policy and change working within the four nations and United Kingdom–wide

So *how* do you gain political acumen and work towards being an 'owl' in your own spheres of influence?

You could attend meetings, as an observer, where colleagues from different parts of the system come together. For example, your organisation's board meeting; other board meetings in your system; the Health and Wellbeing Board; your council's health overview and scrutiny committee; or system partnership meetings or those that bring together health, the local authority, and the voluntary sector. Most of these are possible to attend as a member of the public and many will be webcast. If not, getting in touch with the Chair in advance to explain that you would like to attend for your own personal development should elicit a positive response.

Spheres of Influence

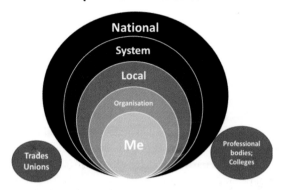

You could approach colleagues in other organisations to spend time shadowing them one-to-one; it gives an opportunity to 'walk in their shoes', understand their drivers and pressures, and build relationships. It also gives them an opportunity to better understand your role and perspective. Think laterally: Could spending time with someone in the council's housing department help you in your role? Or time with the director of adult social care or a social worker, or a local councillor who holds a relevant cabinet portfolio? Might talking to the lead nurse or manager of a care home or shadowing a home carer build your understanding of the challenges they face? If you are a hospital nurse or midwife, how about spending time with a colleague who works in the community and vice versa? What about some conversations with the leaders of your local Healthwatch or voluntary sector coordinating organisation, with leaders of key local charities that work in your area of interest or the Patient Advice and Liaison Service (PALS) in your organisation to get a sense of the public's issues?

All of this activity will take time but will be time well spent in increasing your political astuteness and understanding of the perspectives of others. It will move you from the realms of the 'donkey' and the 'lamb'.

Having Influence and Making Change Happen

So, you've thought about how to become more politically astute and your potential spheres of influence, and so now it is time to think about how you gain influence and make change happen for your patients, for your organisation, and for your profession. Before you start, think through the following:

- What do you want to change and is your message clear? Having a clear message and clarity about what you are looking to achieve/change is vital. Can you explain it in a sentence or a couple of minutes to someone who knows nothing about it? Think 'elevator pitch'.
- Who is the right person to help you progress the thing you want to change? You need to find people who care – really care – about the issue you want to raise or change and you will have much more chance of success. They may 'care' because it's their job, because they are an elected politician and you are a constituent, because

they have personal or professional interest in the issue, or because it is a current issue and resonates as something that merits some use of their time. People are busy and have limited time and brain space, so you need to seek out the people who have a strong reason to care about the issue at hand.

- Once you've identified the person or people who can help you progress your issue, what is their level of understanding of the issue? Are they a generalist or do they understand any special or technical issues you want to progress?

- Is the way you are conveying your message appropriate to the person you are trying to influence in terms of mode, length, level of detail, and technical detail? Do they want short, sharp bullet points, or a detailed and technical briefing? Does it require a face-to-face meeting or can you begin the contact in other ways?

- Is the timing right for a particular discussion/decision/action/piece of work? Are there things going on for the person that you are wanting to influence or engage that might make the timing wrong? Is their financial year at a different stage with different pressures? Do they have staffing/funding constraints? Do they have other, more pressing priorities? Have previous interactions with other nurses and midwives been handled badly so a new approach is needed? Do they feel that they are included at an appropriate stage of discussions or after decisions have been made?

- Who might be opposed to the thing you are trying to change? Is there strong public opposition to the changes that you want to make? If so, you need to increase your conversations and relationship building with those who represent them, be they elected politicians or patient and public pressure groups.

- What are the priorities of the person/people you are trying to influence and how can you align what you want to achieve with their priorities? They will be much more open to your ideas if they also align with their own priorities. Think about what solutions you can offer that also progress their priorities.

- Would it be helpful to bring others with you, particularly groups with whom you have different views, for example patient and carer groups and organisations? There is real power in bringing a wider consortium of people with you to strengthen your case.

- Often within the health sector, we work in hierarchical organisations with 'permission' to act closely controlled. Have you thought about this in connection with the thing you want to achieve and the person you are wanting to influence? Do you have the backing of senior leaders within your organisation and is this even necessary?

Big P Politics

If you want to work more closely and/or influence the thinking and approach of elected politicians, there are a few additional things to consider. We now have a variety of elected politicians across the United Kingdom, from Westminster members of Parliament to devolved Parliament members, from elected city and regional mayors and London Assembly members to a range of councillors working at county, district, unitary authority, and parish council level. If this all sounds like alphabet soup, spending a little time understanding the political system where you live and work is vital, as well as the right person with the power in the right organisation to help with progressing your issue. Starting with your local council's website will help you get a better understanding of the representatives in your area, and who some of the key characters are that make decisions about the issues that you care about and who you may want to influence.

LOCAL AND REGIONAL POLITICS

Having a good understanding of your local politics is essential for nurses and midwives who want to work with colleagues from local government. Many decisions taken by local councillors will directly affect your work, so understanding who forms, implements, has oversight, and gives challenge to the local NHS policy making process is vital.

Thinking about the area where you work, ensure you have a good understanding of:

- The type of local authority(ies) in your area; two-tier (county and district councils) or unitary authority and whether there are parish/borough councils, too. Do you have a directly elected mayor or is the council led by a leader from the majority group? Do you have a regional mayor, too? Some more information about each type of council and their different areas of responsibility can be found on the Local Government Association website (local.gov.uk). This will allow you to think about who is making decisions over the issues that you want to influence.
- Who is in charge politically in your authority(ies)? When are the next elections (some places have annual elections with one-third of councillors elected in rotation; other places have 'all out' elections where all councillors are elected every 4 years)? Are your councils stable politically or does control move from party to party? Your local council(s) website will have this information. This will give you a sense of how close to elections you are; politicians are less likely to make difficult or unpopular decisions when election time is approaching but may be more open to such discussions when they are further away.
- Who are the key people to know? Do you know the names, party affiliations, and interests of key elected members such as the leader, deputy leader, leader of the opposition, cabinet member for health/children/wellbeing/public health, directly elected mayor, chair of the health scrutiny committee/panel, and chair of the health and wellbeing board? Do you know the names and key team members of the leading professional officers who support the elected councillors and who work in areas that are relevant to your role? This could be the director of people/adults and/or children's social care/director of public health. Do you know which other panels/committees they sit on and where they will potentially also have influence?

MPs, PEERS, DEVOLVED PARLIAMENT MEMBERS AND REGIONAL REPRESENTATIVES

Although there is no statutory relationship between local Members of Parliament (MPs), devolved Parliament members, regional politicians, and local councillors, they will often work closely together due to shared interests and constituents in common. However, it would be a mistake to assume that elected politicians from the same party will always work together and, conversely, that those from different parties don't work together. Anything is possible! If there are four nation or United Kingdom–wide policy issues that you would like to influence and change, developing strong relationships with your regional, national, and United Kingdom politicians is essential. Health is often the number one issue in a politician's postbag and inbox, and they will always be keen to have an up-to-date picture of their local NHS.

Thinking about the area where you live/work, ensure you have a good understanding of:

- The names, photos (so you recognise who they are if you meet them!), party affiliations, electoral history, majority, personal, professional and constituency interests, committee, and interest group membership of your local MPs/devolved Parliament members and regional representatives. There may be other MPs whose constituencies are a little further away, but whose constituents also are users of the services your organisation provides and would therefore have an interest. What are they writing about on social media, in the questions they ask in the House of Commons or devolved Parliaments; a search can be made of contributions a particular member has made through the websites listed at the end of this chapter?

- There may be members of the House of Lords, peers, who live locally and who have a particular interest in the services your organisation provides. They can be equally useful people to get to know, despite not having a geographic constituency, and an important local voice.

- If you have a regionally elected mayor, or if you are in London where there are London Assembly members, it is important to get to know who they are and much the same as for the MPs/devolved politicians above, as much background information on them as possible. It is also important to understand the distinct roles they have and where there is cross-over between elected members. For example, if you are working on a service change issue in London, you could need to consult local councillors, London Assembly members (constituency and London-wide members), the mayor of London, local MPs, and London-based peers. In a two-tier authority, it could be parish, district and county councillors, regional mayor, MPs, and locally based peers. In Scotland, Wales, and Northern Ireland where the majority of health issues are devolved, ensure the relevant geographic and subject members are involved.

In summary, if you are wanting to work with, influence, or inform elected politicians, these 10 tips will be helpful:

1. Where does the power lie? Pick who you want to influence carefully.
2. Know your politician; how interested are they in health care and more specifically, the thing you want to change? How do they like to receive info? What are they saying in local/social media? What committees/groups are they on and has it featured in their personal/professional/constituency, majority, electoral cycle?
3. Establish relations in good times; ensure regular contact if appropriate so that if you need to have a difficult conversation, the relationship is already there. Constituents are the most important people to elected politicians, and they will usually give you some time if you are a constituent.
4. Most politicians are generalists dealing with many issues; health is just one of those issues so explain things in a way they can understand.

Laura Moffatt, Member of Parliament for Crawley 1997–2010

Reflections on a Career Change From Nursing Into Parliamentary Politics Then Back to Nursing

My political views were fixed before I started nurse training in 1972.

I completed my nurse education and started work on the wards at Crawley Hospital in 1975, married and had three sons whilst continuing to work on the wards with three short maternity leave breaks.

It was the election of Margaret Thatcher that compelled me into taking my politics more seriously, joining the Labour Party in 1979 and becoming more active in community politics.

Whilst working as a nurse, I was elected to Crawley Borough Council as a councillor in 1984 and held several chair positions and was mayor between 1989 and 1990.

I love nursing and never wanted to do anything else, but there was a tremendous drive within me that is difficult to explain, to want to try and make a greater difference for my community.

After taking the decision to stand as a candidate for Parliament but losing a general election to Nicholas Soames in 1992, I hoped I would be happy to stay with local politics, but no! I decided to have another go for the 1997 general election and was selected on an all-women shortlist for the Crawley seat. The Labour Party saw real value and took every opportunity to promote my nursing background. I was working on the wards as the short campaign started.

On election to the House of Commons, I felt like a fish out of water with no experience of Parliamentary life and really wondered if I had made a terrible mistake. Without the mutual support of the other newly elected, women MPs, the so-called Blair Babes, I could have been overwhelmed.

The first decision I took was to make sure my particular interests were not all NHS or nursing and joined the Defence Select Committee, but I felt strength in the knowledge that I had been working on an NHS hospital ward just a month before.

Soon into my first term in Parliament, the nightmare that any MP faces of a constituency hospital reconfiguration and downgrading of all the major services plan surfaced. It was bad enough to deal with it as the MP, but imagine it being the hospital you trained and worked at as a nurse for 22 years.

My dilemma that I still question myself over is should I have opposed all changes as overwhelmingly as my constituents wanted or tried to understand the reasons behind the proposed changes? As a health worker with an understanding of how safe services should be delivered, for example a maternity unit with fewer than 300 deliveries and dropping, was it responsible to simply object to the proposals to please my constituents?

I chose to engage constructively with the NHS and object where I thought necessary and explain to constituents if I supported a change to NHS services.

It was a hard path to tread, but felt I could not betray decades of a nursing career to be popular and secure reelection.

For most of the three terms (1997–2010) I spent as an MP, hospital reconfiguration was the biggest issue I faced.

Early in my first term while away in Washington with the Defence Select Committee, the chief whip telephoned me to ask if I would like to become a Parliamentary Private Secretary [an unpaid backbench aid to a minister] in the Department of Health, widely seen as a first step on the ministerial ladder. I had no hesitation about turning down the offer. To many, it would be politically foolish, however tempting, but I did not want to be prevented from campaigning or speaking out on issues where I disagreed with the Department of Health. Constituents would have seen it as a betrayal by becoming an 'insider' and I have never regretted that decision.

Being a backbencher, I had the freedom to campaign on issues such as my private members bill on needle stick injury, which was a particular high point in my Parliamentary career as a nurse.

I genuinely feel my nursing background prepared me well for a Parliamentary career. Empathy, organisational skills, and emotional intelligence are all developed as a nurse and are invaluable as a good constituency MP.

After retirement from the House of Commons in 2010, the pull of nursing was too much to resist, so I returned to the most amazing job: nursing.

In a conversation between Catherine Eden and Rt Hon Anne Milton, former MP for Guildford (2005–2019) and a Health Minister, she reflects on some of the skills and approaches that nurses need to be effective at making change happen.

Nurses and midwives have often said to me: 'I don't want to be political'; 'I don't get involved in politics'; 'I'm too busy'; or 'I just want to care for my patients'. But at the same time, they have many valid complaints about their terms and conditions of service, their working environment and how that affects the care they can give, and the organisation for which they work. The misunderstanding arises from the use of the word *politics*. What they mean is they don't want to get involved in *party* politics. They are absolutely right, as the moment they do, they get branded with having an agenda beyond their professional concerns.

I am not sure that nurses and midwives always understand that so much about their working environment and everything about their job is decided within a framework that is decided by politicians. So, like it or not, they are involved in politics. They don't have to get involved in *party* politics, but if they want to get things changed or done, they have to know how to lobby for the changes they want.

Lobbying is a skill nurses should be very good at. Nurses and midwives are good at being agile, adaptive, and reading people well. All the skills that you need to nurse well are the skills that you need to lobby well. We do have the skill set to do it.

Nurses also have the skills to stand in someone else's shoes. For example, if you are a district nurse visiting someone who has rugs all over their house, you know that increases their risk of falling. In order to persuade the older person to get rid of the rugs, it is vital for the nurse to stand in that older person's shoes and understand their concerns about why they don't want to remove all their rugs! Nurses do it every day – we persuade people to do things that they don't always want to do. What you're doing when you are lobbying is trying to persuade politicians and others in position of power to change the things you want to change which the politician might not initially want to do or think is necessary. You have to be able to see things through the political (not party political) lens, but you also have to help them look at things through your eyes and experience. The first question you have to ask yourself is whether you have a compelling case for change, and if you believe you do, why is the minister/civil servant not changing things? You need to understand all the reasons why they're not doing it. As an example, if you wanted to lobby for a reduction in the number of hours nurses work each week, you'd first have to understand the problems that change would cause for the minister. Are there wider implications? If you are only capable of saying the same message over and over again without understanding the barriers, you'll get a headache from hitting your head against a brick wall!

If you're lobbying, notice incremental change. You need to have small goals and staging posts on the way to your end ambition. To use a sailing analogy [my daughter is a professional sailor], if you leave New York and set a course, you only need to alter that course by a fraction of a degree and you'll end up thousands of miles away from where your original course would have taken you. So understand the value of small, incremental changes and congratulate yourself on those small incremental wins – they are all part of the journey to bigger changes.

A lot of time is spent talking about things that are wrong – we all feel better for having a good moan, but don't waste too much time doing it. Agree on what is wrong, agree where you want to end up, and break it down into incremental steps towards the end goal. If you do nothing, nothing will change.

I would also urge nurses and midwives to remain optimistic and not to underestimate the power that you have. You have far more power than you realise. If you have any spare space in your head and time in your day, try and think what you can improve, if not maybe within the lifetime of your career but maybe for those who come after you. I feel very strongly that we all have a responsibility to do that.

5. Evidence-based information is always appreciated; ensure it is concise, appropriate, and relevant.

6. Handle opposition politicians with care, especially around election time and maintain your political and professional independence. Do not get between the dog and the lamppost!

7. Have clear messages, be clear on whose behalf you are speaking, and be clear on what action you want the politician to take.

8. Don't assume they talk to other local politicians – even when in same party. Also, don't assume they will disagree with others in a different political party. Basically, don't assume!

9. Politicians are people. Tell stories about the impact of any changes on constituents, residents, and patients; show projects and invite them to workplaces to see and learn first-hand. It's really powerful and memorable.

10. The photo opportunity. Think about joint opportunities for media activity but always agree between you what you will release.

Nurses Who Became Politicians and Politicians' Reflections on Successful Influencing by Nurses

Becoming a Parliamentarian has long been a career choice for people from a wide range of professions who want to be part of the legislature that makes change happen and potentially be in the ultimate position to influence politics, practice, and professional development. In the history of the modern Westminster Parliament, a small but growing number of nurses have made the leap from caregiver to legislator, giving nurses a crucial voice in Parliament.

The first registered nurse to be elected as an MP was Mary McAlister in 1958. She was elected as a Labour Party MP in the Kelvingrove by-election in Scotland. However, her Parliamentary career was short-lived and she lost her seat the following year.

Other nurses who have followed Mary McAlister into Parliament are Alice Mahon, elected in 1987; Laura Moffatt and Ann Keen, both registered nurses elected in 1997; Anne Moffat, a registered nurse elected in 2001; Jim Devine, a former COHSE registered nurse and UNISON Head of Health, Scotland, was elected along with Anne Milton in 2005. Maria Caulfield was elected in 2015, and Eleanor Smith and Karen Lee in 2017.

Other nurses have entered the House of Lords and have pursued their interest and passion for nursing and health care from their new roles including Baroness Mary Watkins, Lord MacKenzie of Culkein, Baroness Caroline Cox, and Baroness Audrey Emerton.

What Are My Next Steps?

- Start small and build your confidence in influencing for change. Talk to colleagues and nurse and midwifery leaders about changes they have achieved and how they did it. Learning from times when things didn't work out is just as important
- Spend time shadowing someone in your organisation/profession/local system/ nationally who is a person with power to change your issue. They will also learn a lot from you and you will understand more about their competing priorities
- Are there bits of your health and care 'system' that you know less about? How about setting up some shadowing or coffee conversations with colleagues to learn more about the challenges you both face, but from their perspective?
- You may be inspired to think about running to be a local councillor, devolved Parliament member, or an MP – go for it! All the political parties run support and training courses for potential candidates to help and inform you on that journey
- Just do it! But preparation is key; using the steps around identifying the people with power to help, the approach that will be most effective and get your timing right.

Reference

Baddley S., James K., 1987 *Owl, fox, donkey or sheep: Political skills for managers. Manag. Educ. Develop.* 18(1):3–19.

Recommended Further Reading

Florence Nightingale Museum: https://www.florence-nightingale.co.uk.
Local Government Association: https://www.local.gov.uk.
Northern Ireland Assembly: https://www.niassembly.gov.uk.
Scottish Parliament: https://www.parliament.scot.
UK Parliament: https://www.parliament.uk.
Welsh Senedd: https://www.senedd.wales.

CHAPTER 7

The Art and Science of Influencing Change and Measuring Its Impact

Claire Henry ■ Susanna C. Shouls

> *Let us never consider ourselves finished nurses. . . . We must be learning all of our lives.*
> **Florence Nightingale**

CHAPTER OUTLINE

Introduction and Getting Started

This chapter will give you some insights for leading for quality improvement, drawing upon the authors' experiences, the literature, and learning from alumni of the Florence Nightingale Foundation leadership programmes (Florence Nightingale Alumni).

OBJECTIVES

- Understand and describe your opportunity for improvement. Identify your idea/issue/problem and creative solutions.
- Understand the Plan Do Study Act methodology in the context of the model for improvement and 'improvement science'.
- Know how to use quality improvement in your clinical situation as a leader and interpret your learning to create interventions that result in improved outcomes.
- Create practical approaches to conduct tests of change in your setting for your change project.
- Communicate and engage your idea/change project to others, taking their perspectives on board.
- Understand approaches to measuring your change to assess whether it is an improvement.

Importance of Quality Improvement for Health and Care Leaders

> *Every system is perfectly designed to get the results it gets. If we want better outcomes, we must change something in the system. To do this, we need to understand our systems.*
> DON BERWICK, INSTITUTE FOR HEALTHCARE IMPROVEMENT, UNITED STATES

There is global recognition of the importance of quality improvement. The World Health Organization describes it as being 'the action of every person working to implement iterative, measurable changes, to make health services more effective, safe and people-centred' (World Health Organization, 2018). This action requires leadership at all levels.

Leaders are the key influencers of culture and enabling improvements in their organisations (West et al., 2015). Five cultural elements are necessary for sustaining cultures that ensure high-quality, compassionate care for patients:

1. Inspiring visions operationalised at every level
2. Clear, aligned objectives for all teams' departments and individual staff
3. Supportive people management and high levels of staff engagement
4. Learning, innovation, and quality improvement embedded in the practice of all staff
5. Effective team working.

Overall leaders in health care need to be masters of quality improvement methods and be able to lead improvement. Leading quality improvement requires:

- Knowledge: what to do
- Skills: how to do it
- Confidence: 'I can do it'
- Responsibility: ownership and intrinsic motivation
- Belief that you can make a difference
- Continuous learning
- Connection and alignment to other teams/organisations
- Wider support for the improvement

REFLECTIVE LEARNING EXERCISE: WHAT WOULD YOU DO?

Quality improvement in health care is all about making changes with the aim of making health care services better. When faced with a problem or opportunity to make things better, do you:

A. Keep doing what you are doing and hope for different results
B. Try something new and hope this is for the best
C. Apply a thoughtful approach to improve quality
   Hopefully you selected C.
   - Option A is Albert Einstein's description of insanity.
   - Option B is the source of much cynicism. Trying something new can result in improvements, but this is not guaranteed. They often result in change that isn't proven to be better than before, or improvements that are short lived or that have unintended consequences that overshadow any benefits.
   - A thoughtful approach, option C, means those involved and leading change combine the art and science of improvement. The art reflects your approach as an improvement leader and understanding the 'human factors' around change as well as knowing when and how to apply the science and developing attributes such as curiosity and tenacity. The science is the method and associated tools improvement leaders use with rigour and a consistent focus to ensure

that change is demonstrated to result in improvement. Many of the skills you have learnt as nurses and midwives readily transfer to leading quality improvement.

Where Do I Start?

There are a range of different starting points and inspirations or triggers for quality improvement projects. This is highlighted by three Florence Nightingale alumni.
Observing and seeing what we often miss day-to-day:

> I was walking around and I saw a broken blood pressure machine in a room. I wondered, why is this there? Another day I spotted a broken light, sitting in a corner. I wondered if this could affect staff safety? What is happening here? I can't just sit on this. I decided to make this my improvement project.
>
> SHERIN BROWN, 2021

A sentinel event: this could be a complaint, a safety incident, a near miss, or a team concern:

> I work in an acute ward for adult mental health. When patients arrive, they are so unwell that they lack capacity and ability to make decision about their personal property. We had a patient who was wearing his former university's football shirt which he had unfortunately soiled. It got lost in the wash. He was devastated as this shirt was precious to him. I felt so bad for him. I looked into our complaints and found that many related to property. When I talked to my colleagues, I realised that we were being inconsistent about how we managed our patients' property and what was deemed a risk. I felt that this was an important area to improve patients' experience.
>
> HENRY AKALUKA, 2021

Research, new national guidelines, findings from a clinical audit, performance, and patient feedback:

> Research undertaken by the British Association of Parenteral and Enteral Nutrition survey in 2011 found 25% of elderly patients were at risk of malnutrition. We were also concerned with inadequate hydration in the elderly is associated with increased morbidity and mortality. My project was based on this research finding and understanding the opportunities for improvement in my ward were.
>
> SHERRIN JOSEPH, 2021

The commonality of all these three projects is that they have a clear story and all feel worthwhile. They have a very specific starting point, which the alumni make sure is a more general issue in their local context.

REFLECTIVE LEARNING EXERCISE: START AT THE BEGINNING

Take 5 minutes to write down your current improvement ideas in your clinical area. Your ideas could focus on an area you have identified needing to improve (i.e. a problem or issue) or could be a specific idea you feel would result in an improvement (i.e. a solution or intervention).

For example:

- An area needing improvement, a problem or an opportunity: 'We often find we do not have the supplies or equipment we need in the boot (trunk) of our car when we see patients in their own home'.
- A specific idea or a solution or intervention: 'We are planning to design a checklist of equipment and supplies that should be in the book (trunk) of all nurses' cars'.
- Reflect on your notes. If you have jotted down a specific idea, take a few more minutes to describe the problem, issue, or opportunity to make an improvement. This is an important step – there is a risk if you jump to a solution, however good it is, that you will miss the broader opportunity for improvement.

Take a few more minutes to think about how you feel about the area you're planning to improve.

- Is it something you feel passionate about?
- Is it something someone else has asked you to do/suggested needs changing?
- Who benefits? You, patients, their families, other members of the team, other members of staff? More than one group?

What We Mean by Quality Improvement

The term 'quality improvement' can be described as follows:

The systematic use of methods and tools to try to continuously improve quality of care and outcomes for patients and families.

ROSS & NAYLOR, 2017.

This definition suggests a deliberate and focussed effort to make a change which is shown to be an improvement in quality or outcomes. The overall approach supports the identification of various service delivery gaps or opportunities to make improvements, develop solutions, and support the change to address identified gaps and embed and sustain the improvements in quality.

There are six dimensions of quality that will be very familiar to nurses and midwives (Box 7.1). Most quality improvement projects are concerned with more than one dimension. For example, a project by Deepsi Khatiwanda, Florence Nightingale alumni, aimed to:

Promote equality, diversity and inclusion in research engagement/awareness as evidenced by a projected 10% increase in survey uptake amongst Black, Asian and minority ethnic population over an 8-week period.

BOX 7.1 ■ The Six Dimensions of Quality in Health Care

- Safe: avoiding harm to patients and their families that is intended to help them.
- Effective: providing evidence-based care and refraining from providing services that are unlikely to be of benefit.
- Person-centred: establishing a partnership between practitioners and patients to ensure care respects patients' needs and values.
- Timely: reducing waiting times for care and avoiding harmful delays.
- Efficient: avoiding waste
- Equitable: ensuring that care is of the same quality regardless of personal characteristics such as gender, ethnicity, location, or socio-economic status (Institute of Medicine, 2001).

The primary dimension of quality in Deepsi Khatiwanda's project is 'equitable'. The additional dimensions include 'effective', as the research findings will be more generalisable to all patients and also the research approach will be more 'person centred'.

Improving quality of care often results in greater effectiveness and/or efficiency. It can be helpful to understand the logic and use this to get greater buy-in to your ideas. For example, Deepsi Khatiwanda could apply this logic to a specific research study and the potential financial cost of suboptimal research if the research findings are not generalisable to the whole population.

IMPROVEMENT METHODS

Many different improvement models and tools have been developed and used in health services over the years such as Lean (Womack & Jones, 1996), Six Sigma (Bhote, 1989), and the Model for Improvement (Langley et al., 2009). There is no clear evidence that one approach is better than the others. It is more important that there is a systematic approach, consistency, and rigour in its use (Ross & Naylor, 2017). In other words, switching approaches can cause confusion and resentment and may feel like goal posts are continually moving. These methods have their roots in the manufacturing industry, and there are key principles that are common to all:

- Understanding that health care are systems and system thinking.
- Using data to understand variation with the aim to reduce unnecessary variation in processes.
- Giving all staff the opportunity to contribute to and act on ideas for improvement.
- Using multiple testing and trialling as a way to learn and improve.
- Continuing to focus on patients, carers, the public's experiences, and outcomes (Alderwick et al., 2017).

There has been an evolution of theories and approaches that recognise improving health services and public health is complex. A complex adaptive system needs quality improvement methods and leaders that approach problems with many interdependent factors with the intention to enable integrated changes in structures, processes, and patterns (of behaviour and outcome) (Plsek & Greenhalgh, 2001; Sustainable Improvement & Horizons Teams, 2018; Arnold et al., 2018). These approaches build on and all use the key principles described by Alderwick et al. (2017) alongside leadership approaches and insights to work in complex adaptive systems.

THE NHS CHANGE MODEL FOR HEALTH AND CARE

The NHS Change Model (NHS England, 2018) was developed to create a framework and, through this, a common language and approach across the English health care system. This framework cuts across other different models and recognises that health systems are complex.

At the centre of the model (Fig. 7.1) is creating a common shared purpose, which is when a group of individuals align their belief systems or values with a common challenge, vision, or goal. The focus is on the *why*, not the *what* or *how*. The model gives ideas, prompts, tools, and resources that you can use as required when you lead improvements

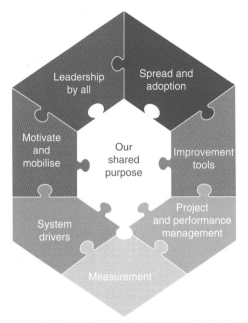

Figure 7.1 The NHS Change Model (NHS England, 2018).

in quality – it gives you a systematic way to consider important dimensions that support the focused aim or shared purpose.

There is also a natural sequence to enable improvements in care.

- Understanding the problem or opportunity for improvement
- Building the will and conditions for change
- Developing clear aim(s) and ideas for change
- Establishing baseline measurement
- Trying out ideas for changes and evaluating if these are an improvement (next to the baseline)
- Implement ideas that have been demonstrated to work
- Spread and sustain the ideas that work

This sequence is not totally linear. As you develop your skills and mastery in practice, you will find that most problems are like the layers in an onion. This means that the process of trialling and testing improvement ideas reveals new areas needing attention. There is also an evolution over time of some of the components. For example, engagement and communication with patients, staff, and teams will develop from initial understanding of the opportunities for improvement to involvement or codesigning ideas for testing and trials in practice to final solutions being embedded into practice.

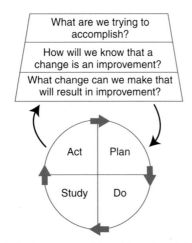

Figure 7.2 The model for improvement (combined figure) (Langley et al., 2009).

MODEL FOR IMPROVEMENT

The model for improvement shown (Langley et al., 2009) is a simple and intuitive method to improve quality of care (Fig. 7.2). It starts out with three fundamental questions:

1. What are we trying to accomplish?
2. How will we know that change is an improvement?
3. What change can we make that will result in improvement?

In order to understand the first question, we must fully understand the opportunities for improvement and create our shared purpose or aim. Once we have a clear aim, then we need to be assured we have a measurement or evaluation approach to know if any changes we make are an improvement or not. The final focus is identifying what ideas and changes we have that we expect to make an improvement.

With this foundation in place, the next step is using 'Plan Do Study Act' cycles of change. This gives you the opportunity to try out ideas without the pressure of assuming they will be adopted. A test of change can be very small, for example testing an idea for the next patient or next clinic, or the test can be large. You use what you learn to inform the next cycle of improvement. At the centre of Plan Do Study Act cycle of change is predicting what will happen in the planning stage, measuring the impact of your idea, and learning from this during the study phase. The final step, Act, is one around decision making – are you adopting, adapting, or abandoning your idea? The scale of the test depends on the phase of your project.

You can use the Plan Do Study Act Cycle of change at all phases of the project: learning (including engaging with stakeholders and developing measurement), testing, and implementing.

For example, take Sherin Joseph's project from earlier (page 3). She works in an elderly care ward and was inspired by a national nutritional study to understand opportunities for improvement in her ward. The aim of this project aim was to 'increase the percentage of recorded food and fluid intake among elderly patients'.

Box 7.2 shows how she used Plan Do Study Act cycles of change to help her to develop her ideas and begin testing her approach.

You can see that the developmental approach Sherin Joseph adopted helped her to lead the project in such a way that the staff, who will ultimately need to adopt any change, helped develop ideas and carry out the tests. This crucial principle increases the chance that the change can be sustained as the approach is more likely to be incorporated into the usual clinical processes.

The common criticism of Plan Do Study Act is that the approach has not been used with rigour, and steps are omitted to get results. As a leader, it is your choice to create the right culture for improvement and leading by example . Being curious and being open to ideas that you feel may not work as well as those you feel will work. Direct people to try things out, create evidence and understand unintended consequence. For example, when Sherin Joseph thought a team member's idea was unlikely to work, she did not stop them from using Plan Do Study Act on the idea but instead directed them to try other ideas at the same time. This created trust and confidence between her and her team..

REFLECTIVE LEARNING EXERCISE: PLANNING YOUR FIRST PLAN DO STUDY ACT CYCLE OF CHANGE

Think about how you could construct an idea into a Plan Do Study Act cycle test of change. The following prompts (Box 7.3) will help you.

The Florence Nightingale alumni found that making a record of their plans and approaches helped them to maximise their learning and be creative. Some of their key learning points from carrying out Plan Do Study Act exercises include the following:

- Team working: It is important to value different skills and highlight the positive contributions each member makes and remember to give constructive feedback in a manner in which you'd like to receive it yourself.
- Observation: Stand back and watch what is really going on – either be that fresh pair of eyes or ask others outside of your team to observe and give new ideas.
- Hidden rules can constrain us and our thinking (e.g. this is how we always do things).
- Reducing variation and improving consistency of performance is an improvement.
- Simple, real-time measurement helps.
- Inclusive involvement: Make sure all those affected by change are involved, including patients and families.

Planning: Understand the Problem and Develop an Aims Statement

Fully understanding the problem or opportunity for improvement and setting your aims statement is an important phase to help you to plan improvements.

There are a number of opportunities for improvement in any clinical service. These can relate to all or some of the dimensions of quality – they can focus the clinical environment; the experiences of patients, families, and staff; how teams work together or with each other; practising new evidence-based care; or ensuring that standards of care are consistently met.

BOX 7.2 ■ **Example of a Series of Plan Do Study Act (PDSA) Cycles of Change by Sherin Joseph, Alumni**

PDSA Cycle	Plan	Do	Study	Act
1.	Establish the baseline by reviewing documentation. Predict there is room for improvement.	Review documentation.	Less than 40% of patients had documented food and fluid intake.	Continue with the project and this measurement approach.
2.	Understand ideas and potential areas for improvement. Predict that this will raise awareness of the problem and give practical ideas.	Talk to ward manager. Talk to other team members.	Patients who have dementia were unable to communicate their needs. Some staff were not aware of documentation.	Focus on patients who are more vulnerable. Need to understand mealtimes. Raise awareness of documentation.
3.	Raise awareness of documentation requirements and learn more about mealtimes. Predict staff will realise the documentation is important.	Share documentation and observe mealtimes every day for a week.	Patients have likes and dislikes. Staff vary in their approach and knowledge of the documentation.	Share observations with the team. Continue to raise importance of documentation.
4.	Clearer allocation of staff to provide more help and record. Predict that documentation and hydration/nutrition improve.	Staff allocated in morning huddle – nurse in charge keeps an eye. Allocated staff help patients choose, eat and drink, and record.	The documentation improved with the greater clarity of staff and which patients are vulnerable.	Combination of 3 and 4 resulted in improvements. Continue with this approach for more days.
5.	Continue to allocate staff to vulnerable patients and note likes and dislikes. Predict staff become more confident.	Allocated staff make sure help choosing, eating and drinking, and recording.	Improvement sustained over a week.	Continue with staff allocation. Focus on sustaining this improvement. Understand potential role of patient's visitors in the future.

> **BOX 7.3 ■ Prompts That Help You to Plan Your First 'Plan Do Study Act' Cycle of Change**
>
> **Plan**
>
> - What are your current questions/theories?
> - What is your prediction?
>
> **Do**
>
> - What do you see? What are the measures?
>
> **Study**
>
> - How did what you see and the measures match your prediction?
>
> **Act**
>
> - What next – what is your decision? Do you adopt your change? Do you adapt? Do you abandon?
>
> ---
>
> Prompts adapted from Williams (2019) Williams, D.M., 2019. Coin Spin PDSA Exercise Facilitator Guide. DMW Austin, Austin, TX.

It can focus on nonclinical systems; back office systems such as staff recruitment, supervision, and finance systems; the layout and environment of clinical areas; and clinical care.

The challenge is often to create focus and realistic goals (Dixon-Woods et al., 2012). A leader who chooses to take an approach that promotes shared construction of the problem and solutions is more likely to develop a sustainable approach. This may require caution and courage to avoid creating 'short-term commotion that quickly becomes part of the noise of competing priorities' (Martin et al., 2019).

Our experience is that curiosity is an important attribute for leaders of quality improvement as is the ability to see the situation from other people's perspectives (i.e. patients, families, colleagues). Having a curious and open mind about why something has or hasn't occurred is key to understanding the root causes. As a leader you can cultivate this in others by how you frame questions and orchestrate enquiry to further understand root causes.

'THE FIVE WHYS' IS A USEFUL TOOL FOR QUALITY IMPROVEMENT LEADERS

By repeatedly asking the question *Why?* you can peel away layers of symptoms, which can lead to the root cause of a problem. Very often the initial reason for a problem will lead you to another question. When using the technique in practice, you may find you need to ask a question fewer or more times than five.

The trick is to use open questions and build on the answers provided. See how far you can go and avoid using easy answers such as 'because we don't have enough staff' or 'because the computer systems are bad'.

Rachel Holmes, a Florence Nightingale alumni, used this approach in her improvement project as shown in Box 7.4. Her project aimed to improve the experience of enhanced observations for adult male inpatients in a secure, forensic mental health unit.

Rachel Holmes' 'five whys' example highlights interrelated themes and starts highlighting areas for potential improvement involving service uses, building protected

> **BOX 7.4 ■ Describing the Problem Using the Five Whys: Enhanced Observations in an inpatient mental health unit**
>
> 1. Enhanced observations are not being carried out effectively. **Why?**
> 2. Staff don't always consider them a vital/fundamental nursing intervention. **Why?**
> 3. Lack of understanding/clarity of rationale/training in meaningful engagement. **Why?**
> 4. Not enough value/emphasis on observations as a protected time rather than a 'tick box' exercise. **Why?**
> 5. Service user is not always involved in the reviews /termination. **Why?**

time into system, consistent training, measuring benefits, and supporting associated practice development.

Most health care system problems are multifaceted and multilayered. By taking the time to be curious and working with staff, she is creating a culture ready for improvement.

The 'five whys' isn't the only tool available to understand the potential root causes of a problem, but it is a helpful tactic for leaders to embrace a culture of curiosity.

Observation and Active Listening

Taking time out to simply observe current care and actively listen to different perspectives is a helpful tactic and will complement other data. When you are immersed within a service or system, it can sometimes be difficult to see things that are obvious to someone outside the system.

When you are trying to improve health care services, you often find that:

- People do not always do what they say they do
- People do not always do what they think they do
- People do not always do what you think they do
- People cannot always tell you what they need
- Things are not always as they seem (NHS III, 2008)

You can walk through a patient journey (Cooper & Henry, 2021), sit in a clinic or observe how people interact with each other in meetings, and see how your intervention works or doesn't work in practice. If you are talking to people as part of your observation, use open questions and be nonjudgemental – aim to see things from their perspectives (staff, patients, carers, visitors). These concepts were originally developed in the design industry (Burns et al., 2006; Cottam & Leadbeater, 2004) and applied to health services.

REFLECTIVE LEARNING EXERCISE: BRAINSTORM WHAT INFORMATION EXISTS ALREADY ABOUT YOUR TOPIC AREA/ OPPORTUNITY FOR IMPROVEMENT

What data and intelligence exists already to help you to understand your opportunity for improvement?

Think about what you know about structure (facilities, equipment, staff), process (diagnosis, treatment, preventative care, patient education and/or inputs), and outcomes (patient/family outcome and experience).

BOX 7.5 ■ Features of a Good Aims Statement

- A worthwhile topic
- Outcome focussed
- Measurable
- Specific population
- Clear timelines
- Succinct but clear

Adapted from Langley, G., et al., 2009. The Improvement Guide: A Practical Approach to Enhancing Organizational Performance, second ed. Jossey-Bass Publishers, San Francisco.

What does it tell you now?

What are the gaps? What and who can help you? Think about any questions you have now. Think about who you could work with to develop your thinking and analytical approaches.

Aim Statement

An aim statement simply describes what you intend to achieve with your project in terms of the outcome rather than solutions or interventions. Your outcome will often describe one or two dimensions of quality described previously (Box 7.5). It answers the question, 'What are we trying to accomplish?' in the Model for Improvement and describes your shared purpose. Aims statements are an important improvement tool for communication and project focus.

When you draft your aims statement, it can be easy to use local jargon and make assumptions about what others understand. It can be helpful to ask people outside of the project

---

BOX 7.6 ■ Reviewing Aims Statement: Practical Examples and How to Make a Good Aims Statement Even Better

Aims Statement	What Is Good	Even Better If/Have You Considered?
To safely move most health visiting face-to-face contact to a virtual platform to ensure safety of the team, the families we look after and the public during the COVID-19 pandemic (Theresa Oseyenum, Florence Nightingale alumni)	Worthwhile topic Clear Clear population (health visiting service)	Could be slightly more succinct Geography of Theresa's team Timescale Clear description of what Theresa means by safety. How will it be measured?
Aim of project is to increase the percentage of recorded food and fluid intake among elderly patients in ward x. (Sherin Joseph, Florence Nightingale alumni)	Worthwhile topic Clear Clear population (ward, elderly)	Included the baseline and ambition Potentially tighter population (patients identified as vulnerable in the elderly care ward)

circle to give you feedback or ask them to describe their understanding. Don't correct them. Take their interpretation at face value – this is your opportunity to explore and refine your description so it is readily understandable to more people. We find that developing measurement alongside your aims statement can help definition, especially if it is open ended. We also find that asking a range of different people can help ensure everyone understands your aim.

The art of giving feedback is an important leadership skill for quality improvement. The Florence Nightingale alumni have found that focussing on the positives and supporting people to consider other options works well. Box 7.6 illustrates how alumni review aims statements.

Further Information

There are a number of other tools available to support a fuller understanding around the opportunities for improvement outlined in Box 7.7. We always recommend working out what information exists already, and Box 7.8 prompts this thinking.

Doing: Change and Improvement – It's All About People

A round man cannot be expected to fit into a square hole right away, he must have time to modify his shape.

BOX 7.7 ■ Approaches to Understand the Opportunity for Improvement

- Mapping the process: create visual picture of how the patient pathway works and associated clinical and nonclinical processes with analysis to identify opportunities for improvement
- Data analysis of experience of patients, families and staff questionnaires, surveys and focus groups (patients, families, staff), experience-based codesign with patients
- Data analysis of the clinical processes and outcome, their patterns, trends, and variation over time (run charts and statistical process control charts)
- Assessment of clinical care against known standards (clinical audit), review of patient records
- Capacity and demand analysis and understanding variation, waiting lists, and waiting times
- Failure Mode and Effect analysis to understand potential route causes
- Pareto analysis (80:20 rule) – a decision-making tool based on finding groups in data that occur most frequently to help you to prioritise effort

---

BOX 7.8 ■ Checking What Data Already Exists

- Patient and staff experience
- Complaints, compliments
- Patient safety incidents
- Service activity data and existing key performance indicators, waiting lists, waiting times
- Existing clinical audits
- National, international studies, and clinical evidence-based guidelines

MARK TWAIN

Doesn't matter who you are or where you come from, the ability to make an impact comes from you.
LEONIE BROWN, FLORENCE NIGHTINGALE ALUMNI

As leaders we need to be mindful of bringing people with us as we lead change. Others can make or break any improvement idea, no matter how good it is in theory. A robust approach to using Plan Do Study Act cycles will help you to give people at the centre of change the opportunity to try out an idea, evaluate the improvements, and build their confidence and belief in shaping what works.

A project by Charlotte Pay (Florence Nightingale alumni) aimed to reduce the levels of anxiety for patients who have autism and are admitted to an acute mental health unit. For Charlotte Pay, working through the Plan Do Study Act cycles in a deliberate and organised way was a significant point of learning. It gave her a greater understanding of the teamwork and leadership styles in the organisation and in the project team. Team members had a lot of existing knowledge and expertise to share. She found that predictions and actions became more realistic (see Box 7.3 for the prompts Charlotte Pay used). The project team also gave her a greater reach across the organisation as they had different contacts and networks. Charlotte's leadership approach had a broader impact – those involved felt recognised and valued with wider potential benefits on staff morale and well-being.

This process taught me how to utilise the skills around me and to make individuals feel appreciated in their contributions. A team can action plans and get results in a way an individual cannot.
CHARLOTTE PAY, 2021

Charlotte's learning highlights the importance of working with clinicians whose practice was at the heart of the change. There are clearly other stakeholders who are important to any improvement project.

You can employ a structured approach to working with others in a project and communicating about a project.

1. Proactive stakeholder management and engagement
2. Project planning: clear plans on how you expect to achieve the aims and action planning

PROACTIVE STAKEHOLDER MANAGEMENT

The primary steps in proactive stakeholder management are as follows:

1. Identify who to involve
2. Prioritise them
3. Understand them
4. Manage them

Many quality improvement projects skip over these steps and only focus on a limited number of stakeholders and approaches for engaging with them. The reasons often feel valid – time is limited or there is an expectation (perceived or real) to start doing things to get results quickly. However, the consequence of not engaging with the right people early on is that things take longer or the potential is simply not realised.

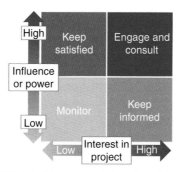

Figure 7.3 Stakeholder power/interest matrix with broad action.

The starting point is brainstorming: Who are your stakeholders? Think of the names you know, job titles, and teams. Then think about how important they are to achieving the goals of your project. There are two dimensions:

- Their influence or power (to achieving the goals of your project)
- The interest they have in your project

This matrix is illustrated in Fig. 7.3, and you can see by using this grid that you have a tactical approach to proactively manage your stakeholders. Remember, different people may be important at different stages of your project.

The next step is to understand your stakeholders and build your focus for this activity on your priorities. Use the following to quickly brainstorm what you know or might deduce about your stakeholders, and be curious to understand them better for the benefit of the project.

- Who are they? (Names/job titles)
- Are they leaders? Cynics? Realists? Optimists? Ambitious? Committed? Because they have to be? Because they want to be? Are they supporters or saboteurs? Or ambivalent?
- What do they hope for?
- Big and small hopes. Do they want the meeting to finish? Do they think the issue is impossible to improve? That there is an easy solution? Do they want recognition? Promotion? What else?
- What do they know?
- About the topic in question? About other topics that might be relevant? What history is there? What experience have they had? What beliefs do they hold? (e.g. failure to meet targets results in punishment). What are their other priorities?
- What do they fear?
- More work. Failure. Soft and fluffy people ('just do it' as a preference). That it won't make any difference. Loss of status. Looking foolish. Admitting they don't know something. Taking risks. The limelight. What else?

Another way to understand stakeholders is to think about personal styles and how they like to work and what may engage them and sustain their engagement. We are all different, and we know that people relate to the world around them in quite distinctive ways. A pragmatic model is that of Merrill and Reid (1999) who describe four personal styles: analyst, amiable, expressive, and driver (Box 7.9).

All four personal styles are important and needed in a team as they all bring different qualities. No one style is better than another. When you look at the styles you may see

---

BOX 7.9   Characteristics of Personal Styles: A Key to Understanding Others

Analyst	Amiable	Expressive	Driver
Analytical	Patient	Verbal	Action-orientated
Controlled	Loyal	Motivating	Decisive
Orderly	Sympathetic	Enthusiastic	Problem solver
Precise	Team person	Gregarious	Direct
Disciplined	Relaxed	Convincing	Assertive
Deliberate	Mature	Impulsive	Demanding
Cautious	Supportive	Generous	Risk taker
Diplomatic	Stable	Influential	Forceful
Accurate	Considerate	Charming	Competitive
Fact finder	Preserving	Inspiring	Determined
Systematic	Trusting	Dramatic	Result-orientated
Logical	Congenial	Optimistic	
Conventional		Animated	

Modified from Merrill, D.W., Reid, R.H., 1999 Personal Styles and Effective Performance: Make Your Style Work for You. CRC Press, London..

---

yourself and also see others. Be careful to not pigeonhole individuals. We may have different preferences in different situations, so in one situation someone could be amiable and in another they may be a driver.

A person may respond to potential change according to their style. There are generalisations about how the different types may respond to change/fear of change described below.

Analytical
>   Not enough information
>   Making the wrong decision
>   Being forced to decide

Driver
>   Loss of control
>   Failure
>   Lack of purpose

Amiable
>   Damaged relationships
>   Confrontations
>   Not being recognised for efforts

Expressive
>   Being ignored
>   Being asked for detail
>   Being linked with failure

Differences in people's styles, skills, and interests are a strength for health and social care teams, and ideally these should be celebrated. It is useful to understand where these differences may cause clashes. Also deal with fears and manage expectations.

When there are differences of opinion or people are less enthusiastic than you are, it can be helpful to step into their shoes to see the world from their perspective. This was the experience of Gerard Jennings, Florence Nightingale alumni:

*As a leader I was keen, passionate, and driven. Reflectively I had to be aware that the passion may
have spilled over into being pushy, wanting people to work at the speed I demanded, so I was aware
to check all emails and my communication approach throughout to be careful of this.*

GERARD JENNINGS, 2021

REFLECTIVE LEARNING EXERCISE: STAKEHOLDERS

Identify your main stakeholders (don't forget to name/label them)
Spend time working the influence/interest matrix: their level of influence or power
  (to help you to achieve the project's outcomes) and their level of interest
Brainstorm some ideas about how you could engage with them
Select a couple of actions you can try out on your next working day

Involved Approach to Creating Aims and Clarity of Approach and Plans

It is easier to engage, communicate, and involve people in projects when there is clarity
over action plans and how everything fits together to achieve the overall aim. There are
two complementary tools that can help.

The first is a driver diagram. A driver diagram is a visual picture that describes the
relationship between the overall aim and those key drivers that influence the outcome
in the project. It outlines this overall logic, and then you note the change ideas you have.
For example, recalling Rachel Holmes' project:

Aim: improve the experience of enhanced observations for adult male inpatients in a
secure forensic mental health unit. The primary drivers were:

Ward environment
Staff involvement and competence
Service user involvement
Documentation

You can see that these drivers will work together and influence the current experience
of enhanced observations in the ward. Generally, it is useful to break down primary drivers
into secondary drivers. For example, secondary drivers for service user involvement were:

Service user understanding of rationale (of enhanced observation)
Service user involved in reviews of their enhanced observation

The final part is simply listing the change ideas. These are the things that you will be
testing, using the Plan Do Study Act cycles of change, to see if and how they work in
practice. Some of Rachel's change ideas were:

Developing a routine satisfaction questionnaire for service users
Creating prompts to be included in the patient safety huddle (including a prompt for
  service user involvement)
Having staff wear an observation badge

Driver diagrams are often called a 'plan on a page', allowing the team to see all the
key influences and ideas in a simple format, and this helps communication around what
is currently being tested and what will be tested in the future. Our experiences are that
driver diagrams are best kept simple and change over the course of a project as the
opportunity for improvement evolves. Remember, the diagrams are a tool, not a master.

Action planning is another helpful tool in quality improvement. It helps keep everyone accountable and communicating around the practical parts of an improvement project at all stages, from understanding the opportunity to sustaining improvements.

Most organisations have project planning templates and methodologies you can follow. Our experience is that working on a 30-60-90 day planning cycle is less cumbersome and creates more realistic plans because quality improvement projects tend to identify new topic areas (remember the onion layers). As you are still learning, it is important to retain flexibility.

Final Reflections

A good intention and aim for action planning is to create a positive momentum of progress – small steps that are achievable build up everyone's confidence towards a collective aim. Remember stakeholders' inputs may need to evolve as your project progresses. Another good intention is to be mindful of their time and ensure engagement is meaningful for all.

There are three final tips for proactive stakeholder management:

1. Always focus on the end point: What do you need your stakeholder to do to help progress the project?
2. Always meaningfully involve those who are directly affected by any changes throughout the project (these are the people – colleagues, other staff members, patients – whose patterns of working or behaviours will be changing)
3. Keep a continuous focus on influential people who can make a difference – other senior leaders to maximise the chance that you receive active support when you need it. Passive support often isn't enough.

Studying: Measurement to Support Improvement

By 1856, Florence Nightingale had transformed hospital care in the Crimean War – her next step was to use statistics to convince the British army and government of the need for widespread reform.

With her mortality diagram, Nightingale wanted MPs and army officials to get a quick visual understanding of the scale of the problem, counteracting their entrenched belief that soldiers died from wounds rather than unsanitary hospitals.

THE SCIENCE MUSEUM, 2018

Measurement and evaluation help you to answer the second question in the model for improvement: 'How will I know that my change is an improvement?' and using measurement to answer the question: 'Is this change an improvement or not?'

The reality is that data, measurement, and analysis touch all phases of any quality improvement project:

- Helping you to fully understand opportunities for improvement and variation
- Prioritising your areas of focus and interventions
- Deciding what ideas work in practice
- Communicating benefits
- Supporting spread and sustainability.

It can be helpful to think of measurement as your honest friend in an improvement project. For example, it will help you to decide as you conduct Plan Do Study Act cycles of change if you need to adopt, adjust, or abandon an idea. It gives rigour to your approach and decision making.

QUANTITATIVE OR QUALITATIVE DATA?

Your project can include quantitative and/or qualitative data. Quantitative data simply describes data that you can count (e.g. time, how often something occurs, temperature, blood saturation, a satisfaction score). Qualitative data is non-numerical descriptive data (e.g. text, video, photographs, audio recordings). You can collect quantitative and qualitative data at the same time (Box 7.10).

Generally, it is useful to include both types of data because quantitative data helps you to know what is happening and the qualitative data gives you an insight into why something is happening.

BOX 7.10 ■ Examples of Quantitative and Qualitative Data and Measurement

	Quantitative	Qualitative
Clinical audit	How often a standard is met Attributes of patients (age, gender) Clinical outcomes	Clinical vignette to describe and inspire (e.g. good practice to replicate or poor practice to help take action)
Reducing waiting times	Waiting times. Data on the process, capacity, demand, activity, and size of the waiting list	Experience and opinions of those waiting Observation of people waiting Observation/photos of waiting room environment
Staff feedback from a training course	Feedback form Levels of confidence Levels of competence Levels of satisfaction, how much they liked the course, etc.	Experiences and opinions expressed in comments Trainers' observation of how people respond and engage Observation of use in clinical practice
Patient and family experience (de Silva, 2013)	Surveys that include questions with a scale (e.g. 1. No confidence; 2. Slight confidence; 3. Moderate confidence; 4. High confidence) The number and type of compliments, complaints	Observation, interviews, comments, focus groups
Resource use	Type of medication/treatment, cost of medication treatment	Clinical assessment of appropriateness

THE SEVEN STEPS TO MEASUREMENT FOR IMPROVEMENT

There is a structured process, available which you can follow to help you to develop measures, that works in parallel to the Model for Improvement. The steps are outlined in Box 7.11 with an example.

What Analytical Skills Do I Need?

As a nurse or midwife, you have core skills in analysis and measurement to provide good care for patients and communicating in a multidisciplinary team. You already use quantitative and qualitative data daily. Think of observing patient's vital signs/other clinical observations: How you know a patient is getting worse or better and how do you use this data to make clinical decisions? What data do you communicate with the team? Measurement for improvement is no different. You have a baseline for which you are making an assessment of improvement. You and the multidisciplinary team use this assessment to inform your decision making.

If you are not a 'numbers person', take 5 minutes and think about why you feel this way. Think about when you use numbers at work or at home and focus on what you can do already. If you feel anxious about numbers, a first step is recognising this and working on your confidence and beliefs (Ma, 1991). You are not alone.

As you apply your existing expertise and your ability to create curiosity and ask questions, focus on working with information analysts. Your insights on clinical processes and providing care are essential to guide their role in quality improvement.

REFLECTIVE LEARNING EXERCISE: GETTING STARTED WITH MEASUREMENT

What Measures Do I Have Already?

Jot down the measures or data you have already next to your aim statement and improvement ideas.

- Do you think they will be specific and sensitive to your change ideas? (Think of your aim statement.)
- Do you have all the three types of measurement?
- Do you have a mixture of qualitative and quantitative data?
- How quickly will you know that your change is an improvement? Will you be waiting hours, days, weeks, or months?

It can be surprising to find out how much data is already available. You can use the seven steps to measurement for improvement to help you to refine your measurement approach.

Developing Measures and an Approach to Evaluating Your Project

As developing measurement is a process itself, it is possible to use the Plan Do Study Act cycle of change to develop and refine your approach to measurement. In the example above you could:

- Test the best way (think *who, what, how, when*) to collect the process measure whether a patient has an expected date of discharge or not.
- Test and work with your informatics department to provide you with robust and timely measures and data.

BOX 7.11 ■ The Seven Steps to Measurement for Improvement			

Step	Measurement for Improvement	What It Means	An Illustration
1	Decide your aim	This is your aims statement.	Our aim is to reduce hospital length of stay in the elderly care wards.
2	Select your measures	Select at least three types: outcome (achieving your aim), process (did the intervention take place), balancing (unintended consequence) This can be a mixture of quantitative and qualitative data.	Outcome: length of stay Process: patient had an expected date of discharge (quantitative) Process: observation of post-take ward rounds (qualitative) Balancing: emergency readmission rate within 30 days Balancing: patient/family feedback on experience of discharge processes (qualitative and/or quantitative)
3	Define your measure	Your measurement description is a bit like a recipe to make sure everyone knows what it means and there is consistency in its construction.	Process measure example: Proportion of patients who had a discharge date set within 24 hours of being admitted to this ward.
4	Collect data	This could involve collecting new data, extracting existing data, or obtaining existing measures from someone.	Length of stay and emergency readmission: from informatics department Expected date of discharge: tally chart when patients are discharged (Use PDSA to develop a practical measure) Experience: Ask for feedback from 10 patients before we start project and 10 patients during the project.
5	Analyse and present	Analysing and presenting the data in a way that makes it easy to make decisions.	Run charts of individual patients' length of stay annotated with changes. Understand themes around patients' feedback.

Continued

BOX 7.11 ■ The Seven Steps to Measurement for Improvement–cont'd			

Step	Measurement for Improvement	What It Means	An Illustration
6	Review your measures	Making decisions based on the data: Do you adopt? Do you adjust? Do you abandon? The improvement idea.	Intervention taking place: Are patients receiving an expected date of discharge? What have we learnt about the new process (having an expected date of discharge)? Or their experience?
7	Repeat steps 4–6	Continue with collecting, analysing, and reviewing.	

As the leader, you will guide what is most practical and robust in any project. A tip is to consider these practicalities as you collect and review your baseline data and keep an eye on the measurement process throughout the project.

Leaders often question how many data points they need for their baseline – this is your measurement before you make any changes. Unfortunately, the answer is often 'it depends'. A simple rule of thumb is at least 10 to 12 data points. However, for some projects you may need many more data points, for example projects that are about improving patient flow, reducing waiting times, and understanding capacity and demand. These projects often need a full understanding of the variation and the nature of variation and are strongly influenced by seasonal, weekly, and daily patterns of working. Your focus is answering the question: 'Is my change an improvement?' Remember, improvement can include a reduction in the variation of process. This is also described as improvement in process reliability.

DISPLAYING DATA OVER TIME USING RUN CHARTS

Displaying numbers over time using a line chart allows you to see patterns in your data. Adding the median – the middle number – to your chart allows you to interpret patterns more precisely and with greater objectivity (Perla et al., 2011).

Imagine that you're tossing a coin – the chance of getting heads for any single toss is 50%. If you were to toss a coin twice, the chance of getting two heads is 25%.

The chance of getting seven heads from seven tosses is less than 1%. In words, it is extremely unlikely to happen by chance alone. We can use these statistical principles to interpret run charts – imagine anything above the line is heads and anything below the line is tails (Box 7.12).

It is more important that you are aware of run charts and that it is possible to use rules to interpret them than remembering the detail. If numbers aren't your thing, develop your understanding sufficiently so you are able to be curious and ask the right questions and work with analysts who can work through the detail.

> ### BOX 7.12 ■ Run Chart Rules
>
> A shift in the process: 7 points or more above or below the median line
> A trend: 7 points or more all increasing or decreasing – these may or may not cross the median line
> An astronomical data point – a data point or two that is dramatically different from the others
> Too many or too few runs
> _____
> Davidge et al., 2017

REFLECTIVE LEARNING EXERCISE: REVIEWING RUN CHARTS

Remembering Sherin Joseph's project with the aim of improving nutrition and hydration in her elderly care ward. She used a key process measure: documenting food and fluid intake in a run chart. The first chart is Sherin's chart, and the second we have created to illustrate a couple of points.

Have the tests of change made an improvement? What else would you like to know? Are these questions you would ask Sherin? Are there questions you would ask a data analyst?

The answer the test of change has made a difference to the improvements in documentation of food and fluid in both graphs.

Using the run chart rules confirms this hunch. Graph 1 is an example of run chart rule 1, and graph 2 is an example of run chart rule 2. An information analyst could help you with this interpretation.

Some reflections for Sherin could be as follows:

Reviewing graph 1: Congratulations! we can see really good progress. It would be interesting to see what the graph looks like after another 7 days to understand the potential level of improvement and what can be sustained. We are curious to learn about the tests of change, staff experience and learning, and future plans. What impact has Sherin Joseph seen on patient outcomes and experience?

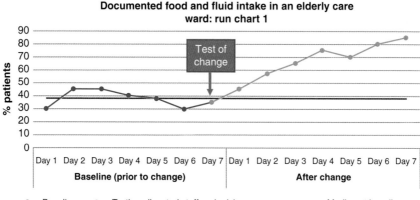

Documented food and fluid intake in an elderly care ward: run chart 1

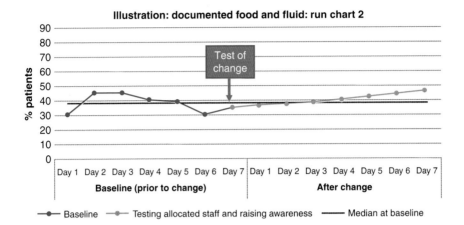

Reviewing graph 2: Congratulations! on the progress, as we can see that there is greater consistency (less variation) in practice, which is a good foundation for further improvement. Curious to learn about staff and patient experience to date and ideas for future tests of change.

You notice the reflections are positive and based on learning and focus on a qualitative understanding.

Acting: Sustainability and Spread: Embedding Your Improvements

Often once the attention and excitement around an improvement project stops, projects do not sustain the same level of improvement. Once you know and have evidence that your proposed changes are an improvement, you need to embed these changes into daily practice. To help this to happen, you will need to build these improved ways of working into existing systems, structures, processes, and habits of teams.

There are approaches that can help you to identify areas to focus on or are at risk of not sustaining improvements. For example, the NHS Sustainability Model is a diagnostic, self-assessment tool to help you to identify areas that may need attention to increase the chance that improvements are sustained. It is useful to obtain a range of perspectives and use the model at an early stage of your improvement project and repeat the exercise a few times during your improvement project. Alongside this, it can be helpful to develop systematic approaches to provide oversight that improvements are sustained with corrective action. This process is called quality control or quality assurance.

Another and complementary area once you have demonstrated improvements is spread. Spread is the process of taking a successful improvement/intervention from a pilot unit or pilot population and replicating that change or package of changes in other parts of the organisation or other organisations. Use the Model for Improvement and Plan Do Study Act cycles of change to support your approach as this will allow appropriate adjustments to be made to fit different and new contexts, including understanding if new areas are ready for change. This approach goes hand-in-hand with sustainability.

REFLECTIVE LEARNING EXERCISE: SUSTAINABILITY

Think about what happens when you or the project lead is on holiday.

Do the improvements stay the same or not? Did people forget, without you there, to remind them? Are you personally involved in actively reminding people to make the change?

If so, the model for sustainability may help you to identify ways to build the change into the daily routines and ways of working.

Summary

This programme is about transformative change; I have transformed personally and professionally. I am enough!

STELLA ESAN, FLORENCE NIGHTINGALE ALUMNI, 2021

Mastery and applying the art and science of quality improvement is essential for health and care services now and in the future. Quality improvement is a critical skill in any leader's armoury. This chapter described the model for improvement with a particular emphasis on the tool Plan Do Study Act cycles of change, which provides the foundations on which to build. Leaders can use Plan Do Study Act to create greater knowledge of the clinical systems, people, and the important measurement to help everyone to answer the question is my change an improvement with the focus on outcome and evidence. As a leader you will continue to learn and develop your quality improvement knowledge and skills, remembering that tools are not the master. Ensure that you do not forget to be curious, flexible, rigorous with your approach and measurement, opportunistic, and tenacious. Know where to focus effort and energy with the ultimate goal to improve health and care for patients, families, and staff.

The world of quality improvement was uncharted territory and involved stepping out of my comfort zone. To seek guidance resulting in built a great rapport with the clinical lead for clinical risk.

STELLA ESAN, 2021

REFLECTIVE LEARNING EXERCISE: GETTING STARTED

Part of this is a personal journey of learning. This is your opportunity to reflect using the following prompts:

How can you use your unique qualities and leadership skills to best enable change that results in improvements? How can you increase your knowledge and practical expertise? We all have to start somewhere. The best way to learn is to try things, reflect, and create supportive networks and seek feedback.

As you start out, our final tips are as follows:

Keep it simple

Ask a friendly colleague

Make a friend (think IT, quality improvement, analyst)

Link with your director or CEO for nursing and midwifery
Start measuring
Plan what you are going to do today

Acknowledgements

Stella Esan
Henry Akaluka
Leonie Brown
Rachael Holmes
Ged Jennings
Charlotte Pay
Theresa Oseyenum
Deepsi Khatiwada
Sherin Joseph

Glossary

Baseline Measurement
The measurement you carry out before you start making changes. This is an essential step. If you don't have a baseline, how do you know you need to make an improvement? It can provide information about where to prioritise effort and learning. It enables you to answer the question, 'Is my change an improvement?'

Improvement Science
Improvement science is a field of study focussed on the methods, theories, and approaches that facilitate or hinder efforts to improve quality.

Lean
Originates from Toyota's 1930 operating model. It is currently described as three step thought process: purpose, process (value stream) and people. In the ideal process, steps are linked by flow, pull and leveling. The emphasis is to ensure processes add value to the customer.

Model for Improvement
Simple framework consisting of three core questions:

- What are we trying to accomplish?
- How will we know a change is an improvement?
- What changes can we make that will result in improvement?

leads to the Plan Do Study Act cycles, which tests small-scale changes, or interventions, to see the effect on outcomes. The quality emphasis is defined by the core questions.

Plan Do Study Act (PDSA) cycles of change
A framework that is part of the model for improvement to create multiple testing and trialling as a way to learn and improve services. The model is based on prediction at the Plan stage, testing at the Do stage, analysis of data at the Study phase, and decision at the Act stage to adapt, adopt, or abandon the idea.

Six Sigma

Improvement framework that focusses on reducing variation in processes to the point that processes are almost defect-free (less than 3.4 defects per million opportunities). It is underpinned by a model called DMAIC (define, measure, analyse, improve, control).

Additional Resources

An Illustrated Guide to Quality Improvement – East London NHS Foundation Trust. https://qi.elft.nhs.uk/qi-illustrations/

Communications in health care improvement – a toolkit. The Health Foundation. https://www.health.org.uk/publications/communications-in-health-care-improvement-a-toolkit.

Design Thinking. IDEO. https://designthinking.ideo.com/.

90-Day Innovation Cycle by the Carnegie Foundation. https://www.carnegiefoundation.org/wp-content/uploads/2014/09/90DC_Handbook_external_10_8.pdf.

Evaluation: what to consider. The Health Foundation. https://www.health.org.uk/publications/evaluation-what-to-consider.

Guide to spread and sustainability. NHS Scotland. https://www.healthcareimprovementscotland.org/about_us/what_we_do/knowledge_management/knowledge_management_resources/spread_and_sustainability.aspx.

Institute for Healthcare Improvement: website of resources. https://www.ihi.org.

Measurement for Improvement (video). Mike Davidge. https://www.youtube.com/watch?v=Za1o77jAnbw.

Measuring Patient Experience. The Health Foundation. https://www.health.org.uk/sites/default/files/MeasuringPatientExperience.pdf.

NHS Elect. Measurement for Improvement Guide: https://www.nhselect.nhs.uk/uploads/files/1/Resource/Service%20Transformation%202016/NHS%20Elect-Measurement%20for%20Improvement-Feb17.pdf.

Quality improvement made simple. The Health Foundation. 2021. https://www.health.org.uk/publications/quality-improvement-made-simple.

Sustainable Improvement Team. 2018. The Change Model Guide. www.england.nhs.uk/wp-content/uploads/2018/04/change-model-guide-v5.pdf.

Survey design. Harvard. https://hnmcp.law.harvard.edu/wp-content/uploads/2012/02/Arevik-Avedian-Survey-Design-PowerPoint.pdf.

Sustainability Model and Guide. NHS Improvement. https://www.england.nhs.uk/improvement-hub/publication/sustainability-model-and-guide/.

The problem with Plan-Do-Study-Act cycles – Reed and Card, 2016. https://qualitysafety.bmj.com/content/25/3/147.

References

Alderwick, H., Charles, A., Jones, B., Warburton, W., 2017. *Making the Case for Quality Improvement: Lessons for NHS Boards and Leaders*. King's Fund, London

Arnold S, et al., 2018. *Health as a social movement*. London: RSA.

Bhote K., 1989. Motorola's long march to the Malcolm Baldrige National Quality Award. *National Productivity Review* 8(4):365–376.

Burns, C., Cottam, H., Vanstone, C., Winhall, J., 2006. *Red Paper 2: Transformation Design*. Design Council, London

Cooper, M., Henry, C., 2021. Walking the Walk: Support for Carers of a Loved One at the End of Life. *Nursing Times* 117 (7), 32–34 [*online*]

Cottam, H., Leadbeater, C., 2004. *Paper 01: Health Co-Creating Services.* Design Council: London NHS Elect; 2017.

Davidge M, Holmes M, Shaw A, Shouls S, Tite M. *Guide to Measurement for Improvement.* London: The Health Foundation; 2017.

de Silva D., 2013. *Measuring Patient Experience: Evidence Scan 18.* The Health Foundation. London.

Dixon-Woods M., McNicol, S., Martin, G., 2012. *Overcoming Challenges to Improving Quality.* The Health Foundation, London.

Institute of Medicine. 2001. *Crossing the Quality Chasm: A New Health System for the 21st Century.* National Academy Press, Washington, D.C.

Langley G, Moen R, Nolan KM, Nolan TW, Norman CL, Provost LP, 2009 *The Improvement Guide: A Practical Approach to Enhancing Organizational Performance.* second edition ed. Jossey-Bass Publishers, San Francisco.

Martin, G., Ozieranski, P., Leslie, M., Dixon-Woods, M., 2019. How not to waste a crisis: a qualitative study of problem definition and its consequences in three hospitals. *Journal of Health Services Research & Policy* 24 (3),

Ma X, 1991. A meta-analysis of the relationship between anxiety toward mathematics and achievement in mathematics. *Journal for Research in Mathematics Education* 20(5):520–540.

Merrill DW., Reid RH., 1999. *Personal Styles and Effective Performance: Make Your Style Work for You.* CRC Press, London.

National Advisory Group on the Safety of Patients in England,. 2013. *A Promise to Learn - a Commitment to Act: Improving the Safety of Patients in England.* Crown London.

NHS England. 2018. *The NHS Change Model Guide*: NHS England.

NHS Institute for Innovation and Improvement (2008) *Through the eyes of ... Observation DVD and card pac*k. SBN: 978-1-906535-30-8

Perla, RJ., Provost, LP., Murray, SK,. 2011. The run chart: a simple analytical tool for learning from variation in healthcare processes. *BMJ Quality & Safety.* 20:46–51.

Plsek, P., Greenhalgh, T., 2001. The challenge of complexity in healthcare. BMJ 323 (625)

Ross S, Naylor C. 2017. *Quality Improvement in Mental Health. King's Fund*, King's Fund, London.

Sustainable Improvement & Horizons Teams, 2018. *Leading Large Scale Change: a Practical Guide.* NHS England, Leeds.

The Science Museum, 2018. *Florence Nightingale: The Pioneer Statistician.* [Online] Available at: https://www.sciencemuseum.org.uk/objects-and-stories/florence-nightingale-pioneer-statistician. Accessed 28 June 2021.

West, M., et al., 2015. *Leadership and Leadership Development in Health Care:* The Evidence Base, first ed. King's Fund, London

Williams DM. 2019. *Coin Spin PDSA Exercise Facilitator Guide.* Austin, Texus: DMW Austin Available at: https://www.davidmwilliamsphd.com/coin-spin-pdsa/. Accessed 03 March 2022..

Womack J., Jones D., 1996. *Lean Thinking: Banish Waste and Create Wealth in Your Corporation*: Simon & Schuster, London.

World Health Organization. 2018. *Improving the Quality of Health Services - Tools and Resources.* WHO. Geneva.

CHAPTER 8

Empowering Nurses and Midwives to Be Digital Health Leaders

Jane Dwelly

> *It's impossible to say whether a hospital is doing its job properly based on haphazardly collected evidence of occasional deaths or mishaps. One needs to compile data that is as complete as possible to see the outcome for the tens of thousands of people who may go through in a year.*
>
> Florence Nightingale

CHAPTER OUTLINE

Digital health has the potential to revolutionise how we care for patients and bring about clinically led change which is truly transformational. Nurses and midwives are well positioned and qualified to support clinical transformation efforts by adopting digital health practices that will result in knowledge-driven care and new delivery models. When nurses and midwives include digital health competencies in their core skills it increases their ability to influence decision making using digital health solutions. This can drive clinical improvements from ward to board and change their organisation's culture to that of a 21st-century health system.

Developing digital competencies enables senior nurses and midwives to become truly transformational leaders in digital health. In turn they are empowered to lead integrated, high-quality care across multiple settings – delivering safe care to patients, saving money, and building deep understanding about population health. These actions realise their organisation's investment in digital health, ensuring that technological solutions meet nursing practice needs and are consistently patient centred.

Adopting digital health competencies into their practice, nurses and midwives will be recognised as leaders in 21st-century health system. In turn they can use these skills to deliver integrated high-quality patient care. Digital health skills are essential and no longer an optional extra. There is no nurse and midwife leadership without digital health.

OBJECTIVES

- Define the digital health skills that are unique to nursing and midwifery.
- Consider the four transformational leadership dimensions in light of digital health competencies.
- Apply digital health outcomes to your leadership practice.
- Build digital health competencies into existing job descriptions.
- Analyse how you can use digital health leadership to transform clinical settings.

Information Makes Every Nurse and Midwife a Digital Health Leader

Think about your day-to-day work as a nurse or midwife. Calculate how many times you collect information about your patient: either by asking them questions, taking observations, or interrogating their patient record. What happens to that information? Sometimes it will be entered into some form of electronic database – a patient administration system (PAS) or an electronic health record (EHR) – in much the same way that paper records were once updated. Some of you will still be using paper records, some of you may have electronic record keeping technology but treat it like a digital paper record, and some of you will work in a fully digital health care setting. This chapter will explore the continuum of digital health as it applies to nurses and midwives. It will make the case for nurses and midwives as key knowledge workers in clinical settings because of the unique conditions created by the fundamentals of nursing and midwifery practice when applied to digital health, and it describes a future state where nurses and midwives are all leaders in digital health transformation.

What do I mean by digital health? The concept has many descriptors including e-health, information and communication technology (ICT), and tech. I use digital health to describe the process of using ICT, computer hardware and devices, software and the cloud, and the collection and analysis of data to improve patient care. Throughout this chapter I will refer to this as digital health. One day, I hope we can drop the adjective 'digital' and just call this activity 'health' as its presence and operation in health care settings will be so unremarkable it won't be seen as a specialism. We are not there yet; however, nurses and midwives have key roles to play now in the development of digital health that will bring about vast improvements to patient care, revolutionise health and care, and change the way we organise our health and care system.

Furthermore, as the largest clinical workforce in all health care organisations, nurses and midwives see the largest number of patients, and these encounters are at all stages of a patient's journey. This mean nurses and midwives are not only able to be present at multiple data points but also have the ability to influence a large patient cadre to use digital health solutions.

Therefore the potential for nurses and midwives to be the conduit for digital health transformation is immense and presents a unique opportunity for nurses and midwives, and those who lead them, at regional and national levels.

In his 2016 report *Making IT Work: Harnessing the Power of Health Information Technology to Improve Care in England*, Professor Robert Wachter made the point that all health care professionals are now practicing in a digital environment and will do so for the rest of their careers. He went on to recommend that NHS staff should receive foundational training in digital information use and integrating digital tools into their practices (Wachter, 2016).

Wachter's well-made points are even more significant in 2021 when the response to the COVID-19 pandemic accelerated the adoption of digital technologies and the use of information across health organisations. This presents a leadership opportunity for senior nurses and midwives, who bridge the gap between the potential of digital health technologies to bring about transformative change, the clinical workforce they lead, and most importantly the patients they care for.

The Impact of Digital Health on Nursing and Midwifery Practice

There is one word that encapsulates the power of digital health to transform patient care: *information*. Health care is 'mostly about information' (Wachter, 2016) and digital health is simply the way of digitalising the collection and use of information to improve patient care.

Digital health is changing how nurses and midwives assess, plan, implement, and evaluate clinical care. As it is integrated in nursing and midwifery practice, it will fundamentally change the way nurses and midwives receive and review diagnostic information, make clinical decisions, communicate, socialise with patients and their relatives, and implement clinical interventions (Rouleau et al., 2017).

Building digital health into nursing and midwifery practice has many benefits, both for patients and nurses. There are five key areas where digital health can improve nursing and midwifery, and therefore nurses and midwives need to develop skills in these areas to bring about these benefits.

PATIENT SAFETY

Digital health provides tools such as barcode medication, e-prescriptions, vital signs monitoring, and discharge reporting. Used correctly, these tools improve accuracy, streamline handovers, and reduce medication errors.

The use of a PAS and an EHR allows nurses to ensure all elements of a patient's care from admission, history, and diagnostics have been recorded and actioned, thereby reducing avoidable errors.

Predictive analytical tools linked to electronic monitoring can alert nurses and midwives to early sepsis or a deterioration in a patient's condition long before it becomes obvious to human observations.

TIME TO CARE

Nurses and midwives build a story of their patients by collecting information about them. Traditionally recorded on paper records and charts, this is a time-consuming practice that needs repeating as the patient moves through care settings and that also builds in the risk of transcribing errors. The physical management of paper records represents a burden to nurses and midwives and decreases efficiency in ward settings. Digital patient records are revolutionary: not only do they allow patient data to be recorded once for all clinicians to see, but they also collect information that contributes to longitudinal databases, thereby increasing knowledge of a population's health needs.

QUALITY CARE

High-quality care, as defined by Lord Ara Darzi in *High Quality Care for All* (Darzi, 2008), is safe and effective care with a positive patient experience. Nurses and midwives can use digital health to carry out enhanced patient monitoring and thus develop highly personal care pathways for individual patients. This results in the most effective treatment being delivered to a patient in the way that works best for them. Ultimately, we will see digital health driving entirely new therapies based on our ability to genetically profile diseases and engineer treatments with pinpoint accuracy.

PATIENT-CENTRED CARE

Digital health tools such as patient-owned diagnostics, tech at home, and monitoring empower the patient by giving them control over their health and decisions about their care. Lifestyle decisions made by patients about using alcohol and tobacco and eating certain foods are improved when the patient is able to focus on outcomes through digital means such as an app on their phone or self-administered electronic diagnostic such as home glucose testing. Qualitative studies of digital consulting have revealed that patient activation to manage their own health leads to increased wellbeing.

THERAPEUTIC ALLIANCES

Digital health changes the clinician-patient dynamic by creating new identities for the nurse or midwife and their patient in which both have a clearly defined and obvious role in improving the patient's health, where possible, or maintaining their quality of life. It has been identified that digital consulting changes the meaning of being a patient and/or a health professional, and the traditional clinician/patient dynamic is reframed in the context of digital consulting into that of a therapeutic alliance (Sturt et al., 2020).

Digital health does not simply make electronic something that was once on paper or in-person, it is a 'cultural transformation of traditional health care' (Meskó et al., 2017). This opportunity was not fully realised until the COVID-19 pandemic made this approach essential to providing continuity of care for millions of patients quarantining at home and had the unintended consequence of delivering a paradigm shift in attitudes to patient-centred care.

Core Elements of Digital Health for Nurses and Midwives

Nurses and midwives are in the unique position of being able to introduce the organisational benefits of digital health while also improving their patients' experience and care. As the pace of this change speeds up there is a risk of developing a two-tier system where some nurses are using digital skills in their practice and others are not. There are lots of reasons for this: organisational culture, previous experience, and bias, and these obstacles present the biggest challenge for digital nurse and midwife leaders.

We see a new paradigm emerging whereby nurse and midwife leaders armed with digital health competencies are positioned to lead and make changes as transformational leaders in health care settings. Indeed, we see nurses and midwives frequently being the link between technology and improved clinical practice. The ubiquity of nurses and midwives in health care settings means they are able to keep lines of communication open as digital health initiatives are being considered, as well as having a significant impact on the development of new digital health systems.

This is evident in three main areas: informatics literacy, technology literacy, and informatics competency. These emerging health care trends are propelling nurses and midwives towards leading health system transformation. The shifts that are taking place align with long-held nursing and midwifery values: a focus on the patient, their safety, and evidence-based care driven by evaluating outcomes.

Let's talk about informatics and how it already informs nursing and midwifery practice. Health informatics is the application of health-related data, information, and knowledge, and nursing informatics is the unique discipline of applying health informatics to patient care. As already discussed, nurses and midwives are knowledge workers and have access to the broadest amount of information about a patient, and the appropriate use of this information, once collected and shared, provides the evidence for transformative improvements in patient care and health system organisation.

Nursing informatics (NI) is defined as a discipline which 'facilitates the integration of data, information, and knowledge to support patients, nurses and other providers in their decision-making in all roles and settings' (Staggers and Thompson, 2002). This definition has been adopted by the American Nurses Association (ANA). It is truly a 21st-century science, and so it is no surprise that nurses spend 50% of their time collecting, coordinating, and documenting information (Haupeltshofer, 2020). NI builds a story around the patient and in doing so improves our knowledge of their health condition and how it can be best treated.

An appreciation of the need for technology literacy naturally follows informatics literacy, and the International Medical Informatics Association (Mantas et al., 2010) has enhanced the ANA definition with the integration of ICT into NI practices. The combination of data collection and analysis when applied through appropriate technology by nurses and midwives leads to a new focus on informatics competency which is defined as having the knowledge, skills, and attitudes to use all three skills in evidence-based nursing care.

Patient care decisions should be supported by timely clinical information gathering the best evidence possible, and nurses and midwives must be able to use informatics and technology to support clinical decision making. Recent work by Natasha Phillips, CNIO at NHSx, has identified a need for an educational strategy to ensure NI is taught at undergraduate level and that current registered nurses and midwives receive in-post training.

Develop Your Professional Leadership Using Digital Health Competencies

The COVID-19 pandemic removed many of the obstacles that were preventing the wholesale implementation of digital health. These were found in organisational culture, a lack of training and confidence in nurses and midwives, and procurement issues. The urgency of the pandemic response removed many of these barriers and we saw how nurses and midwives moved quickly to use digital solutions such as remote consultations to help them care for patients who were quarantining at home. Technologies that patients could use at home to monitor their conditions and record observations were also more widely used and accepted by patients and their families as a core part of care.

In health care organisations, the pandemic response led to nurses and midwives joining ad-hoc interdisciplinary teams made up of other clinicians, managers, and ICT staff to work jointly on emergency measures to provide continuing care. For many, this was the first time that, as nurses and midwives, they had been brought into discussions to provide advice on the appropriateness of a digital health solution from a clinical perspective. This has opened the door for a change in hospital culture, and nurses and midwives should be able to access meetings about digital health if they have not already been invited to participate.

If nurses and midwives are to truly be digital health change agents, then a broader understanding of the hospital or health care setting hierarchy is essential. As we saw during the COVID-19 response, cultural and organisational change is necessary for truly transformative digital patient care.

At all stages of your nurse or midwife career, you can match your clinical experience and skills to a set of competencies in digital health. As digital health skills become ubiquitous to nursing and midwifery practice, these 'specialist' competencies will become mainstream ones and will start to be used in job descriptions, in post responsibilities, and as evidence for revalidation. Therefore any progress in your career will be enhanced by preparation in these areas.

That's the theory. At the time of this writing, a digital health competency framework for nurses and midwives does not yet exist formally in the NHS in England The Australasian Institute of Digital Health (2020) developed and published *National Nursing and Midwifery Digital Health Capability Framework*, and this in turn informed the development of a framework in Northern Ireland and the Republic of Ireland. This approach builds on a focus for the United Kingdom and Ireland Chief Nursing Officer Digital Leadership Group to develop a consistent framework and suite of resources building on the progress of other organisations such as Royal College of Nursing (RCN) to support nurses and midwives to develop digital skills and competence. It also aligns closely with that progressed by Angela Reed during her Nightingale Scholarship in 2017, to define distinct digital capability statements for executive nurse/midwifery leaders as an adjunct to these resources. This work identifies the distinct digital health skills that nurses and midwives need to exhibit at a formative, intermediate and proficient stages of their career. These skills enhance traditional nursing and midwifery areas of practice and are important to focus on as we move forward into an age of increasing digital health care.

For nurses and midwives working in a region that does not have a formal competency framework, the following five career points and associated digital health competencies will be helpful to consider when planning your professional development (Table 8.1).

Update the Four Transformational Leadership Dimensions With Digital Health Competencies

Digital information is a key part of how health organisations, such as hospitals, function. The professional specialism of health informatics concerns the cadre of people, clinical and managerial, who manage the way this information is collected, stored, and analysed. Separately, NI as a specialism is gaining ground as recognition grows about the potential of nursing practice to collect and use information in an evolving digital health system. As digital health has general relevance to all nurse and midwife interactions, it means all nurse and midwife leaders must therefore become leaders of digital health,

TABLE 8.1 ■ Five Career Points and Associated Digital Health Competencies

Informatician	Understands interoperability, data management, and governance
	Understands how information can support nursing decision making
	Can use technology to lead with competence
Change agent	Can develop professional policies to support transformational digital change
	Demonstrates leadership within the organisation to lead digital change programmes
Advocate	Able to align digital health to nursing process
	Collaborate on patient care and technology
Leader	Provide leadership for the adoption and implementation of information systems
Strategist	Ability to design and share a vision of a future digital state that inspires change
	Ability to use technology to support clinical improvement

updating their existing dimensions of leadership to transform health environments into knowledge-led digital health systems.

The Nursing and Midwifery Council (2018) guidance *Future Nurse: Standards of Proficiency for Registered Nurses* presents a context for leadership in the 21st century in which the environment is one of 'continual change, challenging environments, different models of care delivery, shifting demographics, innovation, and rapidly evolving technologies'.

There are two distinct leadership areas that will enable successful digital transformation of the practice of nursing and midwifery. The first is that very senior leaders, such as chief nursing officers (CNOs), need to have the confidence to work with their trust board colleagues to lead a digital health strategy across their whole organisation, especially when a hospital trust is commissioning and implementing an enterprise EHR and the board is signing off a 10-year programme often costing more than £100 million. CNOs may not have training or experience in digital health, but they need to provide specific nursing and midwifery counsel to their board colleagues and directional leadership to their staff with a vision of digital transformation. CNOs will need to be able to articulate the future state that digital health transformation will bring and do so in a way that inspires action.

The second leadership area is the creation of chief nursing information officer (CNIO) and chief midwifery information officer (CMIO) posts. These are key leadership roles for digital transformation and these posts provide an opportunity to broaden a digital strategy into the nursing and midwifery workforce and build strong relationships between IT, clinical, and operations teams.

A CNIO or CMIO working in a large hospital trust should expect to have responsibilities to lead a workforce delivering continually safe and effective high-quality care, in common with all executive clinical leaders. They would also be expected to advocate for and lead on the implementation of information and communication technologies, information collection for decision making, and the development of all nurses and midwives as digital health professionals.

It is clear that existing leadership models do not contain the specific competencies needed to be a nurse or midwife leader of transformative digital health. New models are emerging that allow nurse and midwife leaders to bring about system change using digital health which link NI competencies and advanced leadership skills with the aim of implementing knowledge-driven care (Remus and Kennedy, 2012).

The good news is that there is synergy between the leadership skills needed to manage change and the characteristics identified for enabling digital transformation. For instance, in a recent survey on nurse and midwife-led digital health transformation, the highest scored characteristic was the 'ability to develop appropriate professional and organisational policies to support transformative digital change'. This captures the need for risk management and governance systems across organisations which relate to all change programmes, not uniquely digital ones. Many of the skills needed to bring about digital change are already recognised as general leadership skills, such as change management, leadership, and quality improvement.

When we consider transformational leadership in nursing and midwifery practice, we can see clear alignment with the four elements widely recognised for this approach and competencies successfully used by digital health leaders. A successful digital health implementation in a health care setting also relies on motivating and empowering staff which is the ultimate outcome of transformational leadership.

Being a role model as a digital nurse or midwife leader who uses digital health confidently can be categorised as 'idealised influence', and this a digital health nurse or midwife will encourage colleagues to work to the edge of their practice to adopt innovations.

Describing a future state in which digital health makes patient care safe, efficient, and effective, explaining the benefits of digital health in a way which motivates colleagues and leading teams through large-scale change programmes, is an example of 'inspirational motivation'.

The critical thinking and problem-solving elements of introducing digital health solutions to a health care organisation support 'intellectual stimulation', and the use of digital health networks, mentoring, and learning resources, which are a feature of digital health adoption, relate to the 'individualised consideration' element of transformational leadership.

A Global Perspective

The bicentenary of Florence Nightingale's birth in 2020 will forever be associated with the outbreak of the COVID-19 pandemic: a once-in-a-generation global crisis that claimed more than 3.5 million lives. Nurses and midwives played a critical role in measuring and containing the spread of the virus, and in doing so relied on so many of the infection control lessons identified by Florence Nightingale and which went on to form the basis of modern nursing practice.

Florence Nightingale was also a statistician: if she were alive today, she would be a digital health nurse and a data scientist. She would probably be working on methodologies to evaluate safe, effective, and affordable treatments and clinical innovations to enhance care in the NHS. The way she used information to measure care and drive improvement continues today in digital health nursing and midwifery practice.

It is worth taking a global perspective on nurse-led digital health and looking for international examples of best practice for inspiration. In the United States and Australia, digital health has grown quickly because of economic imperatives associated with payment systems in those countries. The responsibilities of digital nurses and midwives have increased in lockstep with the formal scope of their role supported by digital competency frameworks and professional accreditation.

Conclusion

The potential of digital health to transform the way we organise and deliver patient care is immense. It is also here to stay, and global emergencies such as the COVID-19 pandemic serve to remind us of how essential digital health is in maintaining and extending health services. There is a huge opportunity for nurses and midwives to lead the next stage of the digital health story. Where once we saw digital health solely as the domain of the IT department; this ownership is now shifting to clinicians who are able to lead digital health transformation precisely because of their relationship to the patient. Nurses and midwives are in the unique position of seeing the largest number of patients than any other clinical group and can therefore exert the biggest influence in the shortest period of time.

Nurse and midwife leaders find themselves in the eye of a perfect storm. They can bring about rapid workforce change by building digital health competencies into the job descriptions of every member of their team: from a recently graduated nurse or midwife to a chief nursing or midwifery information officer. This will build confidence in the whole team's outlook when using digital health and support the adoption of a new professional posture for nurses and midwives working collaboratively in interprofessional teams.

References

Australian Institute of Digital Health, 2020. *National nursing and midwifery digital health capability framework* (online). https://www.digitalhealth.gov.au/sites/default/files/2020-11/National_Nursing_and_Midwifery_Digital_Health_Capability_Framework_publication.pdf.

Darzi, A., 2008. *High quality care for all NHS next stage review* (online). https://assets.publishing.service.gov.uk/government/uploads/system/uploads/attachment_data/file/228836/7432.pdf. Accessed 15 May 2020.

Haupeltshofer, A., 2020. Promoting health literacy: What potential does nursing informatics offer to support older adults in the use of technology? *Health Inform.* 26(4) [online]. https://journals.sagepub.com/doi/full/10.1177/1460458220933417. Accessed 6 February 2021.

Mantas, J., et al., 2010. Recommendations of the International Medical Informatics Association (IMIA) on education in biomedical and health informatics (online). https://imiamedinfo.org/. Accessed 23 May 2021.

Meskó, B., et al., 2017 Digital health is a cultural transformation of traditional healthcare. *mHealth.* 3(38) [online]. https://mhealth.amegroups.com/article/view/16494/16602. Accessed 30 January 2021.

Nursing and Midwifery Council, 2018. Future nurse: Standards of proficiency for registered nurses (online). https://www.nmc.org.uk/standards/standards-for-nurses/standards-of-proficiency-for-registered-nurses/.

Remus, S., Kennedy MA., 2012 'Innovation in transformative nursing leadership: Nursing informatics competencies and roles'. *Nurse Leadership.* 25(4) [online]. https://europepmc.org/article/med/23803423. Accessed 28 March 2021.

Rouleau, G., et al., 2017. Impact of information and communication technologies on nursing care: Results of an overview of systematic reviews'. *J. Med. Internet. Res.* 9(4) [online]. http://www.jmir.org/2017/4/e122/. Accessed 5 February 2021.

Staggers, N., Thompson, C.B., 2002. The evolution of definitions for nursing informatics. *J. Am. Med. Inform. Assoc.* 9 (3) [online]. https://www.ncbi.nlm.nih.gov/pmc/articles/PMC344585. Accessed 1 February 2021.

Sturt, J., et al., 2020. How does the use of digital consulting change the meaning of being a patient and/or health professional? Lessons from the long-term conditions young people networked communication study. *Digital Health* 6 (1–13) [online]. https://assets.publishing.service.gov.uk/government/uploads/system/uploads/attachment_data/file/228836/7432.pdf. Accessed 20 September 2020.

Wachter, R., 2016. Using information technology to improve the NHS (online). https://assets.publishing.service.gov.uk/government/uploads/system/uploads/attachment_data/file/550866/Wachter_Review_Accessible.pdf. Accessed 4 January 2021.

CHAPTER 9

Sharing Knowledge and Establishing Expertise Through Writing for Publication

Gemma Stacey

> *Let whoever is in charge keep this simple question in her head (not, how can I always do this right thing myself, but) how can I provide for this right thing to be always done?*
>
> Florence Nightingale

CHAPTER OUTLINE

An aspect of leadership development that is often overlooked by nurses and midwives is sharing knowledge and experience through writing for publication. It is incredibly important to create a commitment to this area of your growth as a leader. Writing for publication is the mechanism for you to gain recognition as an expert in your field, develop networks to extend your practice, and have influence beyond your local environment. Most importantly, it is the tool to share your learning and knowledge of best practice to improve the quality and safety of patient care. By disseminating your practice, you are extending your influence to enable others to replicate or build upon your learning.

There are many excellent resources available which offer a how-to guide on writing for publication. However, we are aware of the numerous blocks and barriers nurses and midwives encounter in their writing process. This chapter will explore the psychological and practical obstacles you may need to confront and provide potential strategies for navigating through the ups and downs of the writing journey.

OBJECTIVES

- Clarify your motivation to write for publication.
- Identify your preferred approach to writing and practically plan to integrate this into your work pattern.
- Develop a working title and identify a potential avenue for publication.
- Reframe the point and process of peer review.
- Explore and address some of the barriers and setbacks you are preempting or have experienced.

Why you should Consider Writing for Publication?

Writing for publication is not an easy task, and there are numerous barriers we encounter as nurses and midwives in putting pen to paper. My suggestion is that you start any writing project by identifying your core motivation to write this particular piece. I suggest this because I have noted through conversations and support I have offered to nurses and midwives that if we focus on the investment of time required to write for publication, then it is unlikely that it will ever become priority. There are always more immediate and pressing demands on our time because of the nature of our working lives. However, if we identify our key motivation to write, we will generate an energy in ourselves which will mean we find the writing process a joy rather than a burden. It can in fact energise us more, so we approach other tasks in our working life with a different level of enthusiasm, perspective, or interest. According to Schwartz and McCarthy (2007): 'Time is a finite resource. Energy is a different story'. They suggest that there are four leadership energies that we should attend to and one of those is our spiritual energy. When we identify how a writing endeavour aligns with our 'human spirit' or 'the energy of meaning or purpose', we feel an imperative to write and it becomes an opportunity which cannot be missed.

We will return to the concept of leadership energies throughout this chapter. Please pause now and take 15 minutes to read the Schwartz and McCarthy (2007) article published in the Harvard Business Review 'Manage your Energy, Not your Time', which can be found at this link: https://hbr.org/2007/10/manage-your-energy-not-your-time.

Establishing Your Motivation to Write

Establishing and exploring your motivation to write should start with the premise that what you have to say is important, and by sharing your knowledge you will have influence on others providing or receiving health and social care. As Florence Nightingale suggested, 'Were there none who were discontented with what they have, the world would never reach anything better'. It is often this discontent that influences the spark in us to investigate, innovate, and thus have a desire to share our knowledge so it can impact others more widely.

REFLECTIVE LEARNING EXERCISE

Table 9.1 shows examples of the factors that are most likely to motivate you to write and also those that may not.

Make a note of all the factors which are motivating you to write. Make this as specific as possible to you and your context. Keep going until you have reached your motivation threshold. This is the point where there are enough drivers for you to have the determination, commitment, and tenacity to write! Now you are ready to think through the *what, who, where, and why*.

When considering your motivation to write, you may find it helpful to explore the following:
- Your key message – *what* knowledge and information do you have a desire to share with others? For example, in a project I undertook exploring how people who use mental health services contribute to the assessment of student nurses, the key

TABLE 9.1 ■ **Examples of Motivators and Demotivators to Write**

Motivators	Demotivators
Have a positive impact on the quality of patient care	My line manager has set this as an objective
Share my work with others who might learn from what I have found	I have seen others do this, and I think I should do it to keep up
Have my work recognised locally, nationally, and internationally	I see this as a huge endeavour that I have to conquer
My work could make a difference to patients and the profession	This is an expectation of nurses and midwives
Build my reputation as an expert in this area	I am likely to be criticised if I don't do this
Network with others who are also passionate about my area	
Start a conversation about what I have learnt	
Improve my CV as I have ambition for a promotion	
I made a commitment to my team and my participants to share this work	

messages I was enthused to share were the potential ethical and power issues that should be taken into consideration before implementing such a process. Having studied the relational dynamics in depth, I felt that it was this key message that could influence how others took this innovation forward.

■ Target audience – *who* do you want to share your knowledge with to have most impact? Does the audience consist of researchers, practitioners, the public, or people who use the services you are working within? This will greatly impact *where* you choose to publish. We will explore the various options later in this chapter, but the factor to consider is how likely is my target audience to read my piece or have access to the publication? For the project described previously, my target audience included professional regulators, clinical educators, and teaching-focused academics. Therefore it was appropriate to publish in a peer review journal which was viewed as reputable and highly regarded among this audience. This gave credibility to my arguments and sparked wider debate and more critical consideration of the initiative. It was also important to present the findings at conferences where these people would attend, to give further opportunity for crucial debate that would also be heard by regulators who were recommending the initiative without this insight or knowledge. Additionally the project was a coproduced endeavour which was undertaken with people who had used mental health services themselves; therefore our experience of undertaking the project in this way was shared at conferences where 'expert by experience' researchers would be in attendance so we could also share our learning of the process as well as the outcome.

■ Desired impact – the *why* question for me is the most important question when exploring our motivation to write. This is the point we ask ourselves why it is essential that we share our learning and our knowledge. It is where we tap into that spiritual energy. For me, this is often about a desire to problematise accepted practice or initiatives so that they are considered from a critical and evidence-based perspective before they are implemented more widely. This is particularly important to me as a mental health nurse with an integral motivation to expose accepted power dynamics and promote shared decision making. It is this internal drive that gives me the fire in my belly and the energy to write. My hope is that I might stimulate a practitioner or educator to reflect on my arguments or reconsider a long-held assumption. For many of my colleagues, the *why* is about ensuring that the best evidence is available to others to drive care standards towards clinical excellence or to share an innovative approach to educating the workforce, which has impacted the confidence and competence of students or practitioners.

REFLECTIVE LEARNING EXERCISE

Take some time now to start to reflect on the *what, who, where, and why* questions. We will revisit each of these throughout the chapter and you should continue to add to these as you read and reflect (Fig. 9.1).

How to Challenge the Inner Critic?

It is important that we actively challenge our inner critical voice so that it does not undermine our confidence and motivation to write. We should start first by exploring the origins of our inner critic. For example, is your belief in your ability to write influenced by a judgement made of you at school around your capability? Do you consider yourself someone who is better at the 'practical' than the 'academic'? Perhaps this is why you pursued a career pathway which has historically celebrated the human attributes of caring over the knowledge and skills required to express care towards others in complex, specialist, stressful, and challenging circumstances. Have you attempted to write in the past and received negative feedback, which has impacted your confidence and made you reluctant to expose yourself to such criticism again? For me, it is all of the above. As a person with dyslexia and a disrupted early education, I have integrated all these critical statements into my thinking patterns. Therefore, I am aware that if I am going to write, I will need to actively challenge my inner critic and develop ways to counter its impact. The following reflective learning exercise will help you to do the same.

REFLECTIVE LEARNING EXERCISE

Make a list of the statements you might hear from your inner critic. Some of the examples I have given may apply to you, but there may also be others. Now provide the

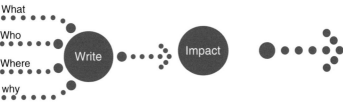

Figure 9.1 Exploring Your Motivation to Write.

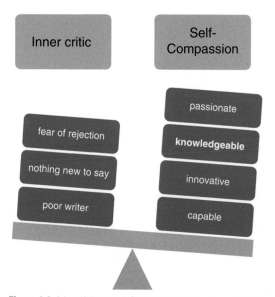

Figure 9.2 Identifying and Challenging Your Inner Critic.

counter argument for this, perhaps the perspective of your most trusted and supportive friend or someone who has always encouraged you to succeed professionally (Fig. 9.2).

By engaging in this activity, you are exercising self-compassion. Evidence tells us that self-compassion is important to enable us to access our creative and original ideas. Our inner critic can induce feelings of anxiety and insecurity, which means our focus becomes narrowed or black-and-white and we feel overwhelmed. Schwartz and McCarthy (2007) explore what they describe as our emotional energy. They recognise that most people perform best when they are feeling positive energy. They suggest that the first step is noticing these negative emotions and the situations which trigger them. You can then engage in rituals such as deep breathing, grounding, or actively changing an environmental stimulus to move out of an anxious state of body and mind. To learn more about the positive effects of self-compassion, please explore the resources available at the following website: https://www.compassionatemind.co.uk/resources/exercises.

Another way of challenging your inner critic is to seek evidence which undermines some of the long-held assumptions you have about your ability to write. Often when we are writing about a topic that we feel extremely passionate about and have a lot of experience in, we get different feedback from when we are marked on an assignment or an examination. It may be that you start your writing journey with a small blog piece that adopts a conversational style and enables you to share your opinion underpinned by your experience and expertise. This is a wonderful way to seek feedback and to receive a reaction to your writing. Alternatively, you may wish to submit an abstract for a poster presentation to conference. This will give you the opportunity to distil your knowledge into a more visual and creative format, which may play to your strengths and preferred approach to sharing and absorbing information. You will be surprised by how many people stop to read your poster, express their interest in your work, and value a conversation with you to learn more. As Florence reminds us: 'So never lose an opportunity of urging a practical beginning, however small, for it is wonderful how often in such matters the mustard-seed germinates and roots itself'.

How to practically Approach writing?

Florence Nightingale said: 'I attribute my success to this: I never gave or took any excuse'. This is applicable to the writing process because for many of us it is seen as an added advantage to our role if we can fit it in when everything else is done (which is never!). There is always an excuse to push writing lower on the priority list. This may be because of the view that writing is primarily about personal career building or CV enhancing. Nursing and midwifery careers are considered altruistic vocations, and therefore to engage in an activity which might be deemed as personally beneficial can raise some feelings of guilt or be in competition to our 'other-oriented' roles. We have already identified that CV enhancement is often not our primary motivation to write; however, we should recognise that increasingly our desire to network and demonstrate our influence beyond our own practice areas is becoming more central to our identity as leaders in health care.

This leads us to thinking about how we can practically protect the time for writing when confronted with multiple demands and competing priorities. Let's start with exploring your individual and preferred approach to writing.

What Is Your Preferred Approach?

- Are you a snacker or do you prefer a feast?
  - This question refers to your preference for short bursts of writing that you engage in regularly to keep momentum and progress going. This is often best scheduled for the time of day when you are least likely to be interrupted and you can give full focus for a short period of time. Alternately, do you prefer to fully immerse yourself in the task at hand for a longer period of time? For example, protecting three consecutive days in your diary to fully engage with the endeavour without the need to switch your attention to other things once you are in a writing 'zone'.
- Can you multitask?
  - Are you able to have several tasks running alongside each other whilst you write? For example, responding to emails at the same time as writing? Many people find this a disruption, but others find it difficult to focus on their writing if they are not aware of what is happening within their main role. So, the ability to maintain engagement is viewed as positive. When considering the 'energy of the mind', Schwartz and McCarthy (2007) suggest that this is counterproductive and that the process of switching attention to other tasks just increases the time taken to complete both tasks. However, I would suggest that this is a preference and we will all have our unique approach.
- Are you distracted by many other jobs?
  - This is otherwise known as procrastinating, that is, the ability to do four loads of washing, cut the grass, and clean the cupboards in the time you have allocated to writing. Traditionally, procrastinating has been seen as a negative trait.

My suggestion is to reframe this as giving you time to think. We shouldn't assume that just because we are not producing words that we are not engaged in the writing process. Sometimes the most creative or crucial point comes to us when we are engaged in routine tasks. It may be that you accept that this will be part of your process and make an effort to make notes around your thought processes that day instead of feeling disappointed with your lack of focus.

- Are you a lone wolf or a social butterfly?
  - This question relates to your preference for writing in isolation or as part of a writing duo or group. The benefits of writing as a social exercise are that you are held to account by others to whom you have made a commitment. Often this involves setting deadlines for each other, and you become incentivised by a feeling of duty to benefit the group. You may meet as a group to decide on the structure of you piece and then allocate sections to individuals or set times when you will write together and benefit from the creativity that can arise from discussion. Alternatively, this prospect may present as a barrier to your concentration and ability to fully focus. You may find more stimulus in the opportunity to think and reflect in isolation if this is where you are able to fully construct your arguments. Whatever your preference, the need to gather feedback on your writing as you progress is always important, so some form of sharing a dialogue should be factored in.
- What does your environment need to look like?
  - Close attention should be paid to the way in which you set up your workspace to enable you to write most effectively. This is very personal but should represent a scenario when you are most likely to be able to access the most creative thinking space. My preference is to be at my desk with all the resources I am likely to need available to me. I enjoy lots of light and warm temperatures so my body is not tense. I do not like to have music or background noise as this interferes with the clarity of my thoughts. I regularly stop to make a drink of herbal tea, which I drink very hot when I am rereading the paragraph I have written. How will you access your most creative thinking space?

REFLECTIVE LEARNING EXERCISE

Now that you have thought about your preferred approach to writing, take a moment to review your diary. How can you prioritise the right kind of time commitment to your

What	is your working title?
Where	are you going to publish?
When	are you going to write?
Who	Will be your writing buddy/mentor?

writing so it becomes an integrated part of your role and receives the same attention as other tasks? Block out the time in your diary and attribute a task to the writing for publication process.

For ideas on how to structure your writing process, see the following resources:

Duffy, S.A., Anderson, J., Barks, L., Cowan, L., Daggett, V., Cristina Hendrix, C., et al., 2017. How to get your research published. International Journal of Nursing Studies. 66, A1–A5. https://doi.org/10.1016/j.ijnurstu.2016.09.002.

Positively Reframing the Process of Peer Review

The peer review process is one of the most challenging aspects of writing for publication. You are voluntarily opening up your work to critique from people who are considered experts in your field. This can feel intimidating and a trigger for the inner critic to raise its voice. Unfortunately, the way in which peer reviewers offer their feedback varies significantly. Many reviewers offer a helpful fresh perspective and come from an informed position. On occasion a reviewer can take umbrage with your writing and their comments can feel extremely demoralising. My key advice is to treat this as opportunity for development as opposed to *criticism*. Our first reaction to a peer review is often defensive. However, if you can think of a peer review as an external and informed perspective on your work which will ultimately enhance its quality, you will receive their feedback as developmental. This is easier said than done though, and it may take a few days and rereads of their comments before you can depersonalise it and really understand their perspective.

If the editor has sent your paper to peer review, they already feel it is of a standard that is appropriate for the journal. That is a huge achievement. If they don't, then it is possible you have not selected the right journal for the focus or type of paper you have submitted, so it is important not to frame this as a rejection.

Below are some top tips for navigating through the peer review process.

1. Engage in informal peer review before submitting:

   Your writing buddy – to gather early and honest feedback, share with a person you feel comfortable showing your raw and unpolished work.

   Your writing mentor – a person who is experienced at writing for publication and can help you shape your paper into an appropriate format for your target audience and publication route.

   Your target audience – a person who represents the audience you are hoping to impact by publishing your work. This offers you the opportunity to check that your points are clear and received as you intend them.

2. Preempt the formal peer reviewers, comments:

   The following are common areas that are picked up by peer reviewers. If you can ensure they are addressed before submitting, you are more likely to get specific and helpful feedback.

   Use recent literature in background/discussion.

   Clearly state what your paper adds to the knowledge base.

   Consider the international relevance/transferability.

   Include ethical considerations even if ethical approval was not required.

3. Points to remember:

   If your paper is rejected, it is probably out of scope for the journal. Use the feedback and submit elsewhere.

   Peer review takes a long time, so do not be disheartened if your paper appears to be sitting in the system with no progress. The editors will be finding the right people to inform their decision.

   Peer reviewers are asked to provide critical feedback for the purpose of developing the paper. Therefore they are likely to be critical as opposed to complementary. As an editor, if I received a peer review which did not identify points for improvement, I would look for a further opinion from an additional reviewer.

   You will have opportunity to respond to the peer reviewers comments. Demonstrate courtesy in your response even if you disagree with the feedback.

   Clearly demonstrate where you have addressed the feedback in your revision.

What are your next steps?

Throughout this chapter we have identified that in order to write for publication, we will need to be intentional about addressing both the psychological and practical barriers we encounter. The next step is to revisit the *what, where, when,* and *who* questions with a different emphasis. This is to move you into action and focus in on your first or next writing endeavour.

REFLECTIVE LEARNING EXERCISE

Use the prompts below to start to formulate your writing plan.

Summary

This chapter has explored and prompted you to consider the following areas:
- Your motivation to write for publication
- Your preferred approach to writing
- The barriers and setbacks you are preempting or have experienced

It has also encouraged you to make practical steps, which will enable you to do the following:
- Integrate writing into your working pattern
- Develop a working title and identify a potential avenue for publication
- Prepare to make the most out of the peer review process

Glossary

- Peer review publication – an article published in a journal or magazine that has been appraised by others who are experts in the same field. It functions to encourage authors to meet the accepted high standards of their discipline and to control the dissemination of research data to ensure that unwarranted claims, unacceptable interpretations, or personal views are not published without prior expert review.

- Blog – a regularly updated online account, typically one run by an individual or small group, that is written in an informal or conversational style.
- Conference abstract – a summary of the main points of your paper/argument that you will present at a conference.

Further Reading

Duffy, S.A., Anderson, J., Barks, L., Cowan, L., Daggett, V., Cristina Hendrix, C., et al., 2017. How to get your research published. *International Journal of Nursing Studies*. 66, A1–A5. https://doi.org/10.1016/j.ijnurstu.2016.09.002.

Schwartz and McCarthy (2007). 'Manage your Energy Not your Time' Manage Your Energy, Not Your Time (https://hbr.org/2007/10/manage-your-energy-not-your-time)

The Compassionate Mind Foundation. https://www.compassionatemind.co.uk/resources/exercises.

Gemma Stacey ▪ Greta Westwood

Throughout this book you have read words of wisdom from Florence Nightingale which have stood the test of time. They feel as relevant today as they did over 100 years ago. As we conclude our book, we would like to encourage you to reflect on some final messages that have come from us, Greta and Gemma, as editors of this book, nurses and executive leaders within the Florence Nightingale Foundation.

Florence encouraged us to 'never lose an opportunity of urging a practical beginning, however small, for it is wonderful how often in such matters the mustard-seed germinates and roots itself'. We hope, now that you have finished this book, several seeds have been planted which will initiate action. By engaging in this material, you have made a practical beginning; however, it is only through conscious and purposeful action that your seeds will grow. What follows are some suggestions of purposeful actions.

Identify, Grow, and Maintain Your Networks

We encourage you to conceptualise networking that centres on relationships, and this should start with your motivation to support a person or organisation by advancing their agenda. By initiating a relationship based on how you can support them, you are demonstrating your value and developing a shared commitment. At a point in the future when this relationship is beneficial for your own agenda, you will be met with generosity and support.

Your networks may be very close and involve frequent and in-depth interaction or can be wide and far reaching. To some extent, your networks will grow organically through the nature of your work revolving around people. However, we also encourage you to be purposeful about the networks you want to build. Requesting an introduction via a colleague, persistently supporting the person's posts on social media, sending an email to introduce yourself and request a meeting, and attending a conference and reviewing the attendee list to identify the people you would like to connect with are all examples of purposeful activities which initiate networks. We must remember that those networks are relationships, and therefore we should frequently think of how to foster them through our communications and actions.

Consider Who Will Be Your Mentor or Coach

At different points in our careers, we will need people who are able to provide us with professional support. This will come in several different forms, but again, we should be purposeful about the nature and focus of the relationship. Two common approaches are mentoring and coaching.

A mentor is a person who sees and knows things you cannot yet see or know yourself because of their experience and expertise. They may have access to networks which are unavailable to you or knowledge that you are still developing because of the time they have worked in the field. This does not presume you are early career leader. Our most senior leaders will still seek mentorship from those more experienced and established in their field, or in a related field. The interaction is often characterised by guidance, education, support, and wise council underpinned by a shared experience of context or role. An additional source of mentorship can come from people in your organisation who are more junior or have a different perspective from you as a result of their ethnicity, age, gender, or sexuality. This is known as reverse or reciprocal mentoring and is based on the wisdom that can be shared from another who holds a different standpoint to yours in the organisation.

A coach is someone who offers you some thinking space to work through the challenges, questions, and assumptions you are encountering. The premise is that you hold the solutions to the challenge within yourself. Through a process of open questioning and reflective thinking, you will work out the most appropriate course of action. Your coach does not need to understand your context or your role, as this person is not advising you on a way forward. Coaching can be extremely empowering and particularly helpful when transitioning to a new leadership role or embarking on a period of organisational change.

An external source of professional support is essential in your commitment to developing self-awareness and emotional intelligence. Both mentorship and coaching can be a unique source of feedback and a rare opportunity to have a metaphorical mirror held up to you so you see yourself from the perspective of someone you trust and respect. Throughout your leadership journey, your focus will change, and this may necessitate a different mentor for an additional stretch or a different approach. It's fine to change – mentors are aware of this, so don't stay loyal to one when really you need to change.

Keep a Close Eye on Your Balance

We often hear reference to good time management as a key skill in leadership. Our suggestion is that you should also pay attention to managing your energy and allocate your time accordingly. It is important to consciously attend to the areas of your life that rejuvenate your energy sources by offering you joy and peace. This may not be as simple as maintaining a good 'work/life balance' as there may well be areas of your work that energise and areas of your personal life which are energy depleting. By paying attention to the impact of day-to-day habits and making a conscious effort to dial up or dial down certain activities, we can become increasingly productive and motivated.

This advice is offered with a note of caution. For some people, work is a life passion and strongly linked to a sense of fulfilment and accomplishment. However, this can lead to a cycle of continuously pushing to do and achieve more, and we may not notice our wellbeing is affected. This is another example where self-awareness and feedback are an important factor. By listening and responding to how others are noticing the impact of your working patterns, you can make conscious decisions about the right balance.

In times of high stress, we can doubt our personal resilience and ability to respond to the demands of our role or the working environment. At these times it is even more important to pay attention to our energy levels as the temptation is to just work harder. It may be that the good habits that maintain your energy have become neglected or replaced by unhelpful behaviours. A good example of this is how we focus our attention. In high-stress periods there is temptation to multitask and respond to many demands simultaneously. The process of constantly switching attention not only negatively impacts our productivity but also impacts on our stress levels and therefore the ability to do our best work. What might be required is a more boundaried approach to allocating time so our full attention can be committed to the task at hand or interaction with others.

At times of high stress, it is easy to blame ourselves for the challenges we are experiencing. As leaders we need to think about how our organisational culture may be perpetuating working patterns that are detrimental to our own and our team's energy levels. Putting in place boundaries around working patterns, sticking to them, and role-modelling them can be a good way to influence a culture which allows people to attend to their energy levels. For example, allowing for planning time in between meetings, encouraging periods away from the screen, and ensuring access to outside spaces have been shown to have very positive impacts on productivity, even in periods of significant organisational change or demand.

Every Part of Your Leadership Journey Will Teach You Something

There are always points in our careers when we find our role or context challenging. We may not be achieving the success we desire or gaining the self-validation which affirms our ability to perform. This could be a result of many factors which can be out of our control or influence; however, we tend to fixate on the poor outcomes and experience low motivation and morale. We encourage you to reframe these situations from the standpoint of a growth mindset or learning always (Clark and Baily, 2018). This perspective focuses predominantly on bringing your hardest and most astute efforts to your work and seeking to improve by learning from whatever transpires.

Research links the growth mindset with many benefits, including greater comfort with taking personal risks and striving for more stretching goals; higher motivation; enhanced brain development across wider ranges of tasks; lower stress, anxiety, and depression; better work relationships; and higher performance levels.

These benefits occur in difficult times because they offer an opportunity to let go of what you can't control and focus your efforts on seeking to improve what you can. It involves creating a psychologically safe culture where mistakes are forgiven and learnt from as opposed to being judged as a failure, a psychologically danger culture. Again, it requires us to exercise our self-awareness and catch ourselves when we judge ourselves, or a colleague, overly harshly. In these moments, there is an opening to explore your reaction and think about how you can use the situation as a point of learning and development.

Ultimately, we can be a highly effective leader and consider ourselves to be a continuous work in progress. The two are mutually dependant as opposed to mutually exclusive. We encourage you to travel curiously; every experience is a learning opportunity and a moment of development.

Don't Look Down. Look Upwards, Sideways, and Outwards

Our final reflection is to remind yourself always of your choices. In the thick of nursing and midwifery leadership there can be a strong draw to focus on the next immediate task or challenge, as there will always be one or many. It can be extremely difficult to look up and consider the multiple options and choices available to you. This is where all our previous advice comes into play:

- Draw upon your networks to ask for a different perspective.
- Seek counsel from your professional support structure to explore your options.
- Engage in activity that maintains your energy and that helps you access your most creative thinking space.
- Give opportunity for yourself and others to learn from failures and see this as a positive contribution to your growth and development.

We wish you the absolute best success in your development as a nursing or midwifery leader and hope you will consider the Florence Nightingale Foundation a source of continuous support at all stages of your career and leadership journey. Every day we learn how to, and develop into, better nurses and midwives, so we leave you with a Florence (1872) quote: 'For us who Nurse, our Nursing is a thing, which, unless in it we are making progress every year, every month, every week, take my word for it we are going back. The more experience we gain, the more progress we can make'.

Further Reading

Clark AM, Sousa BJ. Definitively unfinished: Why the growth mindset is vital for educators and academic workplaces. Nurse Educ Today. 2018 Oct;69:26–29. doi: https://10.1016/j.nedt.2018.06.029. Epub 2018 Jun 30. PMID: 30007143.

Page numbers followed by '*f*' indicate figures, '*t*' indicate tables, and '*b*' indicate boxes.